DORLAND'S
ORTHOPEDICS
SPELLER

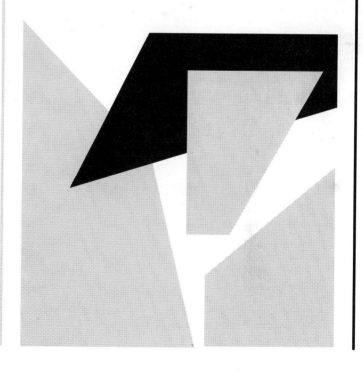

Consultant

SAM W. WIESEL, MD
Professor and Chairman,
Department of Orthopaedic Surgery,
Georgetown University Medical Center,
Washington, DC

Consultant for Syllabication

CAROL A. HART, PhD
Narberth, Pennsylvania

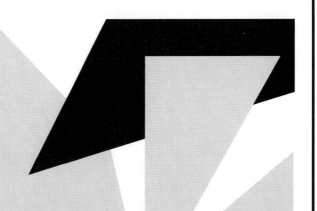

DORLAND'S
ORTHOPEDICS
SPELLER

W.B. SAUNDERS COMPANY
Harcourt Brace Jovanovich, Inc.
Philadelphia London Toronto Montreal Sydney Tokyo

W. B. SAUNDERS COMPANY
Harcourt Brace Jovanovich, Inc.

The Curtis Center
Independence Square West
Philadelphia, Pennsylvania 19106

Library of Congress Cataloging-in-Publication Data

Dorland's orthopedics speller.

p.   cm.

ISBN 0–7216–3752–3

1. Orthopedics—Terminology.   I. W.B. Saunders Company.
 II. Title: Orthopedics speller.   [DNLM: 1. Orthopedics—
 nomenclature.   WE 15 D711]

RD723D67 1993   617.3′0014—dc20

DNLM/DLC   92–13380

Dorland's Orthopedics Speller   ISBN 0–7216–3752–3

Printed in the United States of America

Last digit is the print number: 9   8   7   6   5   4   3   2   1

Preface

The large and growing body of biomedical terminology has long since passed the limit that can be contained in a single volume. The purpose of *Dorland's Orthopedics Speller* is to present a comprehensive listing of terms used in three specialties, orthopedics, physical medicine, and rheumatology, together with a system of acceptable end-of-line breaks. In order to make the book easier to use, multiple listings have been given for hard to find terms, such as eponyms, which will be found not only at the thing named but also at each proper name in the term.

The word list has been compiled from a variety of sources, including the *Dorland's Illustrated Medical Dictionary* database and a number of texts, monographs, and journals. Special attention has been given to eponymic procedures and instrumentation; such terms are extremely common in orthopedics. Care also has been taken to include all terms derived from the official Latin anatomical nomenclature; such terms can be valuable in deciphering the hybrids of Latin and English that are commonly encountered.

DOUGLAS M. ANDERSON
Chief Lexicographer

How This Book Is Arranged

Order of Entries

Dorland's Orthopedics Speller follows the same scheme of arrangement as *Dorland's Illustrated Medical Dictionary*. Main entries follow one another in letter-by-letter alphabetical order regardless of spaces or hyphens that occur within them (see below for special rules for chemical names); compound entries consisting of one or more adjectives and a noun will be found as subentries under the noun. In some cases where there might be a question about where to look to find an entry, entries have been given in more than one place, even under an adjective.

Eponymic terms. Terms containing a proper name are given multiple listings, once under the thing named and once under each eponym. Thus the following entries appear for *Brockman-Nissen arthrodesis:*

> arthrodesis
> Brockman-Nissen a.
>
> Brockman
> B.-Nissen arthrodesis
>
> Nissen
> Brockman-N. arthrodesis

Umlauts are ignored for alphabetization, and proper names beginning *Mc* or *Mac* are alphabetized as though spelled *Mac.*

Chemical prefixes. Italicized chemical prefixes such as the letters *p-* and *o-* and *cis-* and *trans-*, together with numbers, Greek letters, and the small capitals L- and D-, do not count for alphabetization. When prefixes are written out in full, however, as *para-* instead of *p-*, they are counted for alphabetical order.

Subentries

Each subentry appears on a new line following the main entry and is indented. The main entry word in a subentry is represented only by the initial letter, as *cortical b.* under *bone*, with three exceptions. For regular English plurals, the abbreviation is the initial letter followed by 's (as *metatarsal b's* under *bone*). For irregular or Greek or Latin plurals, the entire plural form is written out in full. For possessive forms, the initial letter is followed by 's (as *B's cyst* for *Baker's cyst*). In subentries the main entry word is ignored for alphabetization, as are prepositions, conjunctions, and articles.

Possessive Forms

The use of the possessive in eponyms is controversial. This book follows the example of *Dorland's Illustrated Medical Dictionary*, that is, the 's is favored where the sources for a term justify its appearance. Whether or not to use the possessive form is a matter left to the individual; owing to the present lack of consistency and consensus, no prescription can be given. There are of course some terms in which the possessive is never used, as *Down syndrome*.

Abbreviations and Acronyms

A number of abbreviations and acronyms are given, together with the words or phrases that they stand for. The selection is of course only a small fraction of the abbreviations and acronyms in actual use. If more than one word or phrase is listed with an abbreviation, the terms are given in alphabetical order and each additional term is placed on a new line and indented.

Word Divisions

Acceptable word divisions are given for main entries; syllabication is based on pronunciation. Not all syllable breaks are shown; for example, because single letters at the beginnings and ends of words may not be separated from the rest of the word, such divisions are not given. Likewise, single letters should not be separated from the word elements they belong to in compound words. Breaks that could confuse the reader as to the meaning of a word are to be avoided. In many cases, words may be broken at other places than the ones that appear in this book (for example, different pronunciations imply different word breaks); it is impossible to show every break that could occur for every word. What appears here is one possible system.

Alternative Spellings

A number of words have alternative spellings, ranging from the difference of a single letter to the use of variant forms of Greek and Latin stems. Although every effort has been made to ensure that the spellings included in this book are valid, no indications of preference are given.

Brackets and Parentheses

Some entries require a bit of explanation; these explanations are enclosed in parentheses. Brackets are sometimes used as a part of Latin anatomical nomenclature to enclose an eponym in the genitive case; in this book such eponyms generally appear all lower case (as in *Dorland's Illustrated Medical Dictionary*) but an initial capital for the name is acceptable.

Plurals

Plurals for foreign words, nearly all of them Greek and Latin, are given with the appropriate entries. In addition, they are given again as separate entries if they do not occur within a few lines of the singular form.

Contents

AAA bone

AAOP
American Academy of Orthotists and Prosthetists

Aar·skog
A. syndrome

Aase
A. syndrome

abar·thro·sis

ab·ar·tic·u·lar

ab·ar·tic·u·la·tion

Ab·bott
A. arthrodesis
A. method
A.-Fisher-Lucas arthrodesis
A. and Gill osteotomy

ABC
aneurysmal bone cyst

ABD
abdomen
abdominal

ab·do·men
a. obstipum

ABD (abdominal) pad

ab·duc·tion
Boyes thumb a.
palmar a.
thumb a.

ab·duc·tor
a. digiti quinti
extrinsic thumb a's
lurch a.
a. pollicis brevis
a. pollicis longus
thumb a.

ab·duc·tus
metatarsus a.

Ab·e·nol

ab·late

abrad·er
power a.

ab·scess
arthrifluent a.
bone a.
Brodie's a.
collar-button a.
epidural a.
horseshoe a.
paraspinal a.
paraspinous a.
Pott's a.
psoas a.
serous a.
subaponeurotic a.
subfascial a.
subgaleal a.
subperiosteal a.
subungual a.
syphilitic a.
thecal a.

ab·sence
congenital limb a.

AC
acromioclavicular

A/C
acromioclavicular

acamp·sia

acan·tha

ac·cel·er·a·tion
central a.
linear a.

ac·ces·si·flex·or

Ac·cu·trol

Ace
    acetone

Ace
    A.-Colles fixation device
    A.-Fischer fixation device
    A.-Fischer fixator

Ace ban·dage

Ac·e·phen

Ace·ta

ac·e·tab·u·lec·to·my

ac·e·tab·u·lo·plas·ty

ac·e·tab·u·lum *pl.* ac·e·tab·
  u·li
    sunken a.

acet·a·min·o·phen
    a. and caffeine

ace·tic acid

ac·e·tyl·sal·i·cyl·ic acid

A/C har·ness

Achil·les
    A. bulge sign
    A. reflex
    A. tendon

achil·lo·bur·si·tis

achil·lo·dy·nia
    Albert a.

ach·il·lor·rha·phy

achil·lo·te·not·o·my
    plastic a.

achil·lot·o·my

achon·dro·gen·e·sis
    a. type I
    a. type IA
    a. type II

achon·dro·pla·sia

achon·dro·plas·tic

achon·dro·plas·ty

ac·id
    gammacarboxyglutamic a.
    glacial acetic a.
    hyaluronic a.
    phosphomolybdic a.
    phosphotungstic a.
    polyglycolic a.
    trichloroacetic a.
    uric a.

ac·i·dos·teo·phyte

ac·id phos·pha·tase

ACL
    anterior cruciate ligament

acla·sis
    diaphyseal a.
    tarsoepiphyseal a.

ac·ne·mia

ACP
    acid phosphatase

ac·ro·ar·thri·tis

ac·ro·ceph·a·lo·syn·dac·ty·
  lism

ac·ro·ci·ne·sis

ac·ro·ci·net·ic

ac·ro·con·trac·ture

ac·ro·cy·a·no·sis

ac·ro·dol·i·cho·me·lia

ac·ro·dys·pla·sia

ac·ro·ki·ne·sia

ac·ro·mac·ria

ac·ro·me·ga·lia

ac·ro·me·gal·ic

ac·ro·meg·a·lo·gi·gan·tism

ac·ro·meg·a·loid·ism

ac·ro·meg·a·ly

ac·ro·mic·ria

acro·mio·cla·vic·u·lar

acro·mio·cor·a·coid

acro·mio·hu·mer·al

acro·mi·on
　　Type I, II, III a.

acro·mio·nec·to·my

acro·mio·plas·ty

acro·mio·scap·u·lar

acro·mio·tho·rac·ic

ac·ro·myo·to·nia

ac·ro·my·ot·o·nus

ac·ro-os·te·ol·y·sis

ac·ro·pachy

ac·ro·pachy·der·ma
　　a. with pachyperiostitis

ac·ro·pa·thol·o·gy

acrop·a·thy

ac·ro·sphe·no·syn·dac·tyl·ia

ac·ro·ste·al·gia

ac·ro·syn·dac·ty·ly

acryl·ic

Ac·ta·min

Ac·thar

ac·tin

Ac·ti·no·my·ces

Ac·ti·pro·fen

ac·tiv·i·ty
　　controlled physical a.

ac·to·my·o·sin

adac·tyl·ia
　　partial a.

adac·ty·lism

adac·ty·lous

adac·ty·ly

Adair
　　A. breast clamp

Ad·ams
　　A. forward bend test
　　A.-Oliver syndrome
　　Crawford-A. cup arthro-
　　　　plasty
　　Crawford-A. dexterity test
　　Horwitz and A. arthro-
　　　　desis

ad·ap·ta·tion
　　biomechanical a.
　　therapeutic a.

adap·ter
　　sealing fluid a.

Ad·dis
　　A. test

Ad·di·son
　　A's keloid

ad·du·cent

ad·duct

ad·duc·tion
　　Bunnell thumb a.
　　Edgarton-Grand thumb a.
　　Royle-Thompson thumb a.
　　thumb a.

ad·duc·to·ca·vus

ad·duc·tor
　　a. magnus

ad·duc·tus

ad·e·no·car·ci·no·ma
　　acinar a.
　　acinous a.
　　papillary a.
　　polypoid a.

ad·e·no·ma
　　basophil a.
　　basophilic a.

ad·he·sion

ad·he·sive
    bandage a.

ADI
    atlantodens interval

ADL/PDLS
    activities of daily living/
        physical daily living
        skills

ADP-glu·ta·thi·one

adre·no·cor·ti·coid
    glucocorticoid a's

Ad·son
    A. cerebellum retractor
    A. maneuver
    A. periosteal elevator
    A.-Beckman retractor
    A.-Beckwith retractor

ad·vance·ment
    Codvilla V-Y a.
    ligament a.
    ligamentous a.
    tendon a.
    vastus medialis a.
    Wagner tendon a.

ad·ven·ti·tia

Ad·vil

AE
    above elbow

Aero·Bid

AFB
    acid-fast bacteria

AFO
    ankle-foot orthosis

A-frame or·tho·sis

A/G
    albumin-globulin (ratio)

age
    TW$_2$ bone a.

agen·e·sis
    lumbar a.
    sacral a.

agent
    nonsteroidal anti-inflam-
        matory a.

AGF
    angle of greatest flexion

ag·gre·gate
    proteoglycan a.

A/G (albumin-globulin) ra·tio

AHSC (Arizona Health Science
    Center-Volz) el·bow pros·
    the·sis

aid
    extension a.

aide
    physical therapy a.

ain·hum

air·cast
    a. brace
    a. walking brace

air-splint

Ait·ken
    A's classification of epi-
        physeal fractures

AK
    above knee

AKA
    above-knee amputation

AK amp
    above-knee amputation

Ak·bar·nia
    Campbell and A. proce-
        dure

Akin
    A. procedure

ala *pl.* alae
    a. ilii
    a. of ilium
    alae lingulae cerebelli
    a. ossis ilii

ala *(continued)*
    sacral a.

al·a·nine ami·no·trans·am·i·nase

al·a·nine trans·am·i·nase

alb

Al·bee
    A. graft
    A. hip arthrodesis
    A. lumbar spinal fusion
    A. shelf procedure

Al·bers
    A.-Schönberg disease

Al·bert
    A. achillodynia

Al·bright
    A's disease
    A. hereditary osteodystro-
        phy
    A's syndrome
    A. and Chase arthroplasty
    A.-McCune-Sternberg syn-
        drome
    McCune-A. syndrome

al·bu·min

al·co·hol
    reagent a.

al·do·lase

Al·ex·an·der
    A's view

al·fa·cal·ci·dol

Al·ge·sal

al·go·dys·tro·phy

align·ment
    anatomic a.
    bony a.
    classical a.
    a. of fracture fragments

Al·ka-Bu·ta·zol·i·din

Al·ka·bu·ta·zone

al·ka·line phos·pha·tase
    a.p. serum

Al·ka-Phen·yl·bu·ta·zone

al·kap·ton·uria

Alk PO₄ tase
    alkaline phosphatase

Al·len
    A. maneuver
    A's test

Al·lis
    A. clamp
    A. maneuver
    A. sign

al·lo·ar·throp·a·thy

al·log·e·nous

al·lo·graft
    pelvic a.
    revascularized a.

al·loy
    cobalt-chromium a.
    metal a.
    multiphase a.
    titanium a.

Alou·ette
    A. amputation

ALP
    alkaline phosphatase

ALRR
    arthroscopic lateral reti-
        nacular release

ALS
    amyotrophic lateral sclero-
        sis

ALT
    alanine transaminase

Al·ta
    A. titanium reconstruction
        plate

alu·mi·na

Al·vine
   A. total ankle replacement

am·bi·dex·trous

am·bo

am·bon

am·bu·la·tion

AMC to·tal wrist ar·thro·plasty

AMD
   arthroscopic microdiskectomy

AME bone growth stim·u·la·tor

ame·lia

Amer·i·can Acad·e·my of Or·tho·tists and Pros·the·tists

Amer·i·can Or·thot·ic and Pros·thet·ic As·so·ci·a·tion

Amer·sol

Am·i·ge·sic

am·i·ka·cin

Am·i·kin

Ami·no·fen

Am·i·paque

AML to·tal hip re·place·ment

Amoss
   A. sign

am·phi·ar·thro·di·al

am·phi·ar·thro·sis

am·phi·di·ar·thro·sis

amp·i·cil·lin

Am·pi·cin

am·pu·ta·tion
   above-elbow (AE) a.
   above-knee (AK) a.
   Alanson's a.
   Alouette's a.
   Anderson's a.
   aperiosteal a.
   arm a., complete
   arm a., partial (lower ⅓)
   arm a., partial (middle ⅓)
   arm a., partial (upper ⅓)
   Batch a.
   Béclard's a.
   below-elbow (BE) a.
   below-knee (BK) a.
   Berger's a.
   Bier's a.
   bloodless a.
   Boyd's a.
   Bunge's a.
   Callander's a.
   Carden's a.
   Carne a.
   carpal a., complete
   carpal a., partial
   central a.
   chop a.
   Chopart's a.
   cinematic a.
   cineplastic a.
   circular a.
   closed a.
   coat-sleeve a.
   a. in contiguity
   a. in continuity
   cutaneous a.
   definitive a.
   Dieffenbach's a.
   double-flap a.
   Dupuytren's a.
   eccentric a.
   elliptic a.
   end-bearing a.
   Farabeuf's a.
   fish mouth a.
   flap a.
   flapless a.
   Forbes a.

am·pu·ta·tion *(continued)*
forearm a., complete
forearm a., partial (lower ⅓)
forearm a., partial (middle ⅓)
forearm a., partial (upper ⅓)
forequarter a.
Gordon-Taylor a.
Gritti's a.
Gritti-Stokes a.
guillotine a.
Guyon's a.
Hancock's a.
Hey's a.
hindquarter a.
hip a., complete
interilioabdominal a.
interinnominoabdominal a.
intermediary a.
interpelviabdominal a.
interscapulothoracic a.
interscapulothoracic forequarter a.
intrapyretic a.
Jaboulay's a.
kineplastic a.
King and Steelquist a.
Kirk's a.
Kutler a.
Langenbeck's a.
Larrey's a.
Le Fort's a.
leg a., complete
leg a., partial (lower ⅓)
leg a., partial (middle ⅓)
leg a., partial (upper ⅓)
levels of a.
linear a.
Lisfranc's a.
Littlewood a.
long AE a.
long AK a.
long BE a.
long BK a.
lower-third AE a.

am·pu·ta·tion *(continued)*
lower-third AK a.
lower-third BE a.
lower-third BK a.
Mackenzie's a.
Maisonneuve's a.
major a.
Malgaigne's a.
mediotarsal a.
medium AE a.
medium AK a.
medium BE a.
medium BK a.
metacarpal a.
metacarpal a., complete
metacarpal a., partial
metatarsal a., complete
metatarsal a., partial
mid-third AE a.
mid-third AK a.
mid-third BE a.
mid-third BK a.
minor a.
mixed a.
Morestin a.
musculocutaneous a.
oblique a.
open a.
osteoplastic a.
oval a.
Pack a.
partial foot a.
partial hand a.
pelvic a., complete
periosteoplastic a.
phalangeal a., complete
phalangeal a., partial
phalangophalangeal a.
Pirogoff's a.
Pollock a.
primary a.
provisional a.
racket a.
ray a.
rectangular a.
Ricard's a.
secondary a.
semicircular flap a.

am·pu·ta·tion *(continued)*
    short AE a.
    short AK a.
    short BE a.
    short BK a.
    shoulder a., complete
    Sorrondo Ferré a.
    Spittler and McFaddin a.
    spontaneous a.
    Stokes' a.
    subastragalar a.
    submalleolar a.
    subperiosteal a.
    Syme's a.
    tarsal a., complete
    tarsal a., partial
    Teale's a.
    tertiary a.
    thigh a., complete
    thigh a., partial (lower ⅓)
    thigh a., partial (middle ⅓)
    thigh a., partial (upper ⅓)
    through-knee a.
    a. by transfixion
    transmetatarsal a.
    transverse a.
    traumatic a.
    Tripier's a.
    upper-third AE a.
    upper-third AK a.
    upper-third BE a.
    upper-third BK a.
    Vladimiroff-Mikulicz a.

am·pu·tee

Am·spa·cher
    A. and Messenbaugh osteotomy

Am·stutz
    A. resurfacing procedure
    A. total hip replacement
    A. and Wilson osteotomy

am·y·loi·do·sis
    skeletal a.

amyo·pla·sia
    a. congenita

amy·os·the·nia

amyo·to·nia
    a. congenita

amyo·tro·phia
    neuralgic a.
    a. spinalis progressiva

amyo·troph·ic

amy·ot·ro·phy
    neuralgic a.

am·y·ous

AMZ an·tero·lat·er·al dis·place·ment os·te·ot·o·my

An·a·cin

anal·y·sis *pl.* anal·y·ses
    free-body a.
    gait a.
    motion a.
    roentgen stereophotogrammetric a.

Ana·met·ric un·con·strained de·vice

an·apoph·y·sis

An·a·prox

an·ar·rhex·is

an·as·to·mo·sis *pl.* an·as·to·mo·ses
    end-to-end a.
    end-to-side a.
    microvascular a.
    precapillary a.

Ana·tom·ic hook

Ana·tom·ic II hook

anat·o·my
    surgical intervention a.

An·cef

an·chor
    Mitek II a.
    suture a.

an·chor plate

an·co·nad

an·con·ag·ra

an·co·nal

an·co·ne·al

an·co·ne·us

an·co·ni·tis

an·co·noid

An·der·son
    A. procedure
    A. and D'Alonzo classifica-
        tion (of odontoid frac-
        tures)
    A. and Hutchins procedure
    Boyd and A. procedure

an·dro·gen

ane·mia
    Fanconi's a.
    sickle cell a.

an·es·the·sia
    local a.

an·eu·rysm
    popliteal artery a.

an·eu·rys·mor·rha·phy

ANF
    antinuclear factor

Ang·hel·es·cu
    A. sign

an·gi·na
    cervical a.

an·gi·og·ra·phy
    spinal a.

an·gi·om·a·tous

an·gio·sar·co·ma

an·gle
    acromial a.
    acromial a. of scapula
    Alsberg's a.
    Baumann's a.
    Böhler's a.
    capital epiphysis a.
    carrying a.
    CE (center edge) a.
    Cobb a.
    Codman a.
    collodiaphyseal a.
    congruence a.
    costovertebral a.
    a. of declination
    elevation a.
    external a. of border of
        tibia
    external a. of scapula
    Hilgenreiner a.
    a. of inclination
    infrasternal a. of thorax
    internal a. of tibia
    Konstram a.
    kyphotic a.
    lateral a. of border of tibia
    lateral a. of humerus
    lateral patellofemoral a.
    lateral a. of scapula
    lateral talometatarsal a.
    Laurin a.
    lumbosacral a.
    lumbosacral joint a.
    medial a. of humerus
    medial a. of scapula
    medial a. of tibia
    Merchant a.
    Mikulicz's a.
    neck shaft a.
    Pauwels a.
    pelvic femoral a.
    a. of pelvis
    pelvivertebral a.
    Q a.
    quadriceps a.
    radiolunate a.
    rib vertebral a.
    sacrohorizontal a.

an·gle *(continued)*
   sacrovertebral a.
   slip a.
   sternoclavicular a.
   subscapular a.
   sulcus a.
   theta a.
   a. of torsion
   a. of trunk rotation
   tuber a.
   x-ray a.

an·gu·la·tion
   a. of fracture

an·gu·lus *pl.* an·gu·li
   a. acromialis
   a. inferior scapulae
   a. infrasternalis thoracis
   a. lateralis scapulae
   a. lateralis tibiae
   a. medialis scapulae
   a. medialis tibiae
   a. superior scapulae

an·iso·dac·ty·lous

an·iso·dac·ty·ly

an·iso·me·lia

an·iso·sthen·ic

an·kle
   a. arthrodesis
   deck a's
   tailors' a.

an·ky·lo·dac·tyl·ia

an·ky·lo·poi·et·ic

an·ky·losed

an·ky·lo·sis *pl.* an·ky·lo·ses
   bony a.
   extracapsular a.
   false a.
   fibrous a.
   intracapsular a.
   ligamentous a.
   spurious a.
   true a.

an·ky·lot·ic

AN-MDP

an·nu·lar

an·nu·lus *pl.* an·nu·li
   a. fibrosus
   a. fibrosus disci interverte-
      bralis

Ano·col

anom·a·ly
   congenital a. of vertebrae
   Poland's a.

an·os·teo·pla·sia

an·os·to·sis

An·said

An·spach
   A. 65K instrumentation

An·spor

an·tag·o·nist
   associated a's
   direct a's

an·te·bra·chi·um

an·te·flex·ion

an·ter·i·or

an·ter·i·or·iza·tion

an·tero·me·di·al·iza·tion

an·te·ver·sion

an·ti·bi·ot·ic
   a. bead

an·tic·ne·mi·on

an·ti·po·dag·ric

an·ti·spas·tic

an·ti·strep·tol·y·sin
   a. O

Ant·ley
   A.-Bixler syndrome

Anu·phen

AO
  ankle orthosis

AO Fixateur Interne

AO plate

AO/ASIF fem·o·ral dis·trac·tor

AO/ASIF lag screw

AOPA
  American Orthotic and Prosthetic Association

AP
  anteroposterior

Apa·cet

ap·ar·thro·sis

ap·a·tite

Apert
  A's syndrome

aper·tu·ra *pl.* aper·tu·rae
  a. pelvis inferior
  a. pelvis [minoris] inferior
  a. pelvis [minoris] superior
  a. pelvis superior

ap·er·ture
  inferior a. of minor pelvis
  spinal a.
  superior a. of minor pelvis

apex *pl.* apex·es, api·ces
  a. capitis fibulae
  a. ossis sacri
  a. of patella
  a. patellae
  a. of sacrum

apha·lan·gia
  complete a.
  partial a.

ap·i·cal

apio·ther·a·py

APLD au·to·mat·ed per·cu·ta·ne·ous mi·cro·dis·kec·tomy

Ap·ley
  A. test

Apo-Am·pi

Apo-Ci·met·i·dine

apo·dia

Apo-Di·clo

Apo-Doxy

Apo-Ibu·pro·fen

Apo-In·do·meth·a·cin

apo·kam·no·sis

Apo-Me·tro·ni·da·zole

Apo-Nap·ro-Na

Apo-Na·prox·en

apo·neu·rec·to·my

apo·neu·rol·o·gy

apo·neu·ror·rha·phy

apo·neu·ro·sis *pl.* apo·neu·ro·ses
  abdominal a.
  bicipital a.
  a. bicipitalis
  clavicoracoaxillary a.
  crural a.
  epicranial a.
  falciform a. of rectus abdominis muscle
  femoral a.
  a. of insertion
  intercostal aponeuroses, external
  intercostal aponeuroses, internal
  a. musculi bicipitis brachii
  a. of occipitofrontal muscle
  palmar a.
  a. palmaris
  plantar a.
  a. plantaris
  Sibson's a.
  subscapular a.

apo·neu·ro·sis *(continued)*
    a. of superior surface of le-
    vator ani muscle
    supraspinous a.
    temporal a.
    vertebral a.

apo·neu·ro·si·tis

apo·neu·rot·ic

apo·neu·rot·o·my

Apo-Phen·yl·bu·ta·zone

apoph·y·sa·ry

apoph·y·se·al

apoph·y·se·op·a·thy

apoph·y·ses

apoph·y·si·al

apo·phys·i·ary

apoph·y·sis *pl.* apoph·y·ses
    basilar a.
    odontoid a.
    a. ossium

apoph·y·si·tis

Apo-Pi·rox·i·cam

apo·plas·mat·ic

Apo-Ra·ni·ti·dine

Apo-Sul·fa·meth·ox·a·zole

Apo-Sul·fa·trim

Apo-Sul·in

Apo-Tet·ra

ap·pa·rat·us *pl.* ap·pa·rat·
us, ap·pa·rat·us·es
    Calandruccio compression
    a.
    a. ligamentosus colli
    locomotor a.
    spine a.

ap·pen·dix *pl.* ap·pen·di·ces,
ap·pen·dix·es

ap·pen·dix *(continued)*
    ensiform a.
    xiphoid a.

ap·po·si·tion
    a. of fracture

ap·proach
    anterior a.
    anterior/posterior a.
    anterolateral a.
    dorsal a.
    extraspinal a.
    intraspinal a.
    lateral a.
    lateral peripatellar a.
    McFarland a.
    midline a.
    posterior a.
    quadriceps turn-down a.
    Radley, Liebig, and
      Brown a.
    retroperitoneal a.
    Senegas a.
    Smith-Peterson a.
    surgical a.
    transabdominal a.
    transoral a.
    transsternal a.
    vastus medialis a.
    volar a.

APR (Anatomic Porous
    Replacement) pros·the·sis

aprax·ia

APTT
    activated partial thrombo-
    plastin time

arach·no·dac·tyl·ia

arach·no·dac·ty·ly
    contractural a., congenital
    (CCA)

arach·noid

arach·noid·itis

Ar·a·len

arch
  anterior a. of atlas
  axillary a.
  bony a.
  coracoacromial a.
  costal a.
  deep palmar arterial a.
  femoral a., superficial
  fibrous a. of soleus muscle
  a's of foot
  hemal a.
  inguinal a.
  Langer's axillary a.
  longitudinal a. of foot
  neural a.
  neural a. of vertebra
  palmar a.
  palmar arterial a.
  popliteal a.
  posterior a. of atlas
  pubic a.
  a. of pubis
  a. of ribs
  subpubic a.
  superficial palmar arterial
    a.
  supraorbital a. of frontal
    bone
  tendinous a. of lumbodor-
    sal fascia
  tendinous a. of soleus
    muscle
  transverse a. of foot
  a. of vertebra
  vertebral a.

ar·cu·a·tion

ar·cus pl. ar·cus
  a. anterior atlantis
  a. iliopectineus
  a. inguinalis
  a. pedis longitudinalis
  a. pedis transversalis
  a. posterior atlantis
  a. pubicus
  a. pubis
  a. tendineus
  a. tendineus fasciae pelvis

ar·cus (continued)
  a. tendineus musculi solei
  a. vertebrae
  a. vertebralis

Ar·drey
  Vidal-A. fixation device

area pl. areae, areas
  Cohnheim's a's
  intercondylar a's of tibia
  a. intercondylaris anterior
    tibiae
  a. intercondylaris posterior
    tibiae

Ar·i·zo·na uni·ver·sal leg
  sup·port

arm
  bird a.
  C-a.
  dead a.
  glass a.
  golf a.
  linebacker's a.
  tackler's a.

Arm
  arm amputation

Ar·my re·trac·tor

Ar·my-Na·vy re·trac·tor

Ar·nold
  A. brace
  A.-Chiari syndrome

ar·rest
  epiphyseal a.

ar·ter·itis pl. ar·ter·it·i·des
  granulomatous a.
  necrotizing a.

ar·te·ry
  a. of Adamkiewicz
  anterior tibial a.
  axillary a.
  brachial a.
  carotid a.
  common digital a.

ar·te·ry *(continued)*
    deep femoral a.
    digital a.
    digital a. of foot
    dorsal digital a.
    dorsalis pedis a.
    femoral a.
    genicular a.
    gluteal a.
    highest genicular a.
    inferior gluteal a.
    obturator a.
    perforating a's
    peroneal a.
    popliteal a.
    posterior tibial a.
    profundus a.
    radial a.
    segmental a.
    subclavian a.
    superior gluteal a.
    tibial a.
    ulnar a.
    vertebral a.
    volar digital a.

ar·thrag·ra

ar·thral

ar·thral·gia
    patellofemoral a.
    a. saturnina

ar·thral·gic

ar·threc·to·my

ar·threm·py·e·sis

Ar·threx grasp·ing stitch·er

ar·thri·fuge

ar·thrit·ic

ar·thrit·i·des

ar·thri·tis *pl.* ar·thrit·i·des
    acute a.
    acute gouty a.
    acute rheumatic a.
    acute suppurative a.

ar·thri·tis *(continued)*
    atrophic a.
    bacterial a.
    Bekhterev's a.
    blennorrhagic a.
    chronic inflammatory a.
    chronic villous a.
    climactic a.
    cricoarytenoid a.
    crystal-induced a.
    a. deformans
    degenerative a.
    degenerative a. of knee
    exudative a.
    fungal a.
    a. fungosa
    gonococcal a.
    gonorrheal a.
    gouty a.
    hemophilic a.
    hypertrophic a.
    infectious a.
    inflammatory a.
    juvenile a.
    juvenile chronic a.
    juvenile rheumatoid a.
    menopausal a.
    monoarticular a.
    a. mutilans
    mycotic a.
    neuropathic a.
    a. nodosa
    a. pauperum
    peripheral a.
    polyarthralgia-a.
    posttraumatic a.
    proliferative a.
    psoriatic a.
    reactive a.
    rheumatoid a.
    rheumatoid a., juvenile
    rheumatoid a. of spine
    septic a.
    a. sicca
    suppurative a.
    syphilitic a.
    trapeziometacarpal a.
    tuberculous a.

ar·thri·tis *(continued)*
   uratic a.
   a. urethritica
   venereal a.
   vertebral a.
   viral a.

ar·throc·ace

ar·thro·cele

ar·thro·cen·te·sis

ar·thro·cha·la·sis
   a. multiplex congenita

ar·thro·chon·dri·tis

ar·thro·cla·sia

ar·throc·la·sis

ar·thro·cli·sis

ar·thro·de·sia

ar·thro·de·sis
   Abbott a.
   Abbott-Fisher-Lucas a.
   Albee hip a.
   ankle a.
   Baciu and Filipiu a.
   Badgley a.
   Blair a.
   Bosworth a.
   Brett a.
   Brittain a.
   Brockman-Nissen a.
   Campbell a.
   Carroll a.
   cervical a.
   Chandler a.
   Charnley a.
   Charnley and
     Henderson a.
   Chuinard a.
   Chuinard and Petersen a.
   compression a.
   Davis a.
   Dunn-Brittain triple a.
   elbow a.
   extra-articular a.
   finger a.

ar·thro·de·sis *(continued)*
   Gant hip a.
   Ghormley a.
   Gill a.
   Gill-Stein a.
   Haddad-Riordan a.
   Henderson a.
   Hibbs a.
   hip a.
   Horwitz and Adams a.
   intraarticular a.
   John C. Wilson a.
   Key a.
   Kickaldy and Willis a.
   Kling a.
   knee a.
   Kuntscher modified a.
   Lucas and Murray a.
   Marcus, Balourdas,
     Heiple a.
   Moberg a.
   Muller a.
   Nalebuff a.
   Potenza a.
   Potter a.
   Putti a.
   Schneider a.
   Seddon a.
   shoulder a.
   sliding a.
   sliding ankle a.
   Smith-Petersen a.
   Stamm a.
   Staples a.
   Steindler a.
   Stewart and Harley a.
   Stone a.
   subtalar a.
   triple a.
   Trumble a.
   Watson-Jones a.
   White a.
   Wickstrom a.
   Wilson a.
   wrist a.

ar·thro·dia

ar·thro·di·al

ar·thro·dyn·ia

ar·thro·dys·pla·sia

ar·thro·em·py·e·sis

ar·thro·en·dos·co·py

ar·thro·erei·sis
   subtalar a.

ar·thro·fi·bro·sis

ar·thro·gram
   injection a.

ar·throg·ra·phy

ar·thro·gry·po·sis
   congenital multiple a.
   a. multiplex congenita

ar·thro·ka·tad·y·sis

ar·thro·klei·sis

ar·thro·lith

ar·thro·li·thi·a·sis

ar·thro·lo·gia

ar·throl·o·gy

ar·throl·y·sis

ar·thro·men·in·gi·tis

ar·throm·e·ter
   KT-1000 a.

ar·thron·cus

ar·thro·neu·ral·gia

ar·thro·no·sos

Ar·thro·pan

ar·thro·path·ia
   a. psoriatica

ar·thro·path·ic

ar·throp·a·thol·o·gy

ar·throp·a·thy
   chondrocalcific a.
   crystal-induced a.
   dialysis a.

ar·throp·a·thy *(continued)*
   facet a.
   HLA-27–positive a.
   inflammatory a.
   osteopulmonary a.
   psoriatic a.
   pyrophosphate a.
   static a.
   syphilitic a.

ar·thro·phy·ma

ar·thro·phyte

ar·thro·plas·tic

ar·thro·plas·ty
   adjusted cup a.
   Albright and Chase a.
   AMC total wrist a.
   Aufranc cup a.
   Austin Moore a.
   Bateman a.
   bipolar a.
   Brigham unicompartmen-
    tal a.
   capsular a.
   Carroll and Taber a.
   cemented total hip a.
   Charnley a.
   Charnley's hip a.
   Christiansen a.
   Crawford-Adams cup a.
   a. cup
   cup a.
   Curtis a.
   double cup a.
   Eaton's implant a.
   Eaton-Littler a.
   excisional a.
   fascial a.
   flexible wrist a.
   Fowler a.
   hip a.
   hip resurfacing a.
   ICLH double cup a.
   implant a.
   implant resection a.
   Indiana conservative re-
    surfacing hip a.

ar·thro·plas·ty *(continued)*
  interpositional a.
  low-friction a.
  Lubinus a.
  metacarpophalangeal joint
    a.
  Meuli a.
  Oxford unicompartmental
    a.
  palmar self-a.
  Paltrinieri-Trentani a.
  proximal interphalangeal
    joint a.
  resection a.
  resectional a.
  resurfacing a.
  revision a.
  St. George sledge knee a.
  salvage a.
  silicone implant a.
  Smith-Peterson cup a.
  Steffe a.
  surface replacement a.
  Swanson a.
  THARIES resurfacing a.
  Thompson a.
  total ankle a.
  total articular replacement
    a. (TARA)
  total hip a.
  total knee a.
  total shoulder a.
  total wrist a.
  trapezium implant a.
  Tupper a.
  uncemented ceramic dou-
    ble cup a.
  Vainio a.
  volar shelf a.
  Volz a.
  Wagner a.
  Wagner resurfacing hip a.

Ar·thro·por I ac·e·tab·u·lar
  cup

Ar·thro·por II ac·e·tab·u·lar
  cup

ar·thro·py·o·sis

ar·thro·rheu·ma·tism

ar·thro·ri·sis

ar·thro·scle·ro·sis

ar·thros·co·pist

ar·thros·copy

ar·thro·sis
  a. deformans
  facet a.
  patellofemoral a.

ar·thros·te·itis

ar·thros·to·my

ar·thro·syn·o·vi·tis

ar·throt·o·my
  hip a.

ar·thro·trop·ic

ar·thro·xe·ro·sis

ar·throx·e·sis

ar·ti·cle

ar·tic·u·lar

ar·tic·u·late

ar·tic·u·lat·ed

ar·tic·u·la·tio *pl.* ar·tic·u·la·
  ti·o·nes
  a. acromioclavicularis
  a. atlanto-axialis lateralis
  a. atlanto-axialis mediana
  a. atlantoepistrophica
  a. atlanto-occipitalis
  a. calcaneocuboidea
  a. capitis costae
  a. capitis humeri
  articulationes capitulorum
    costarum
  articulationes carpi
  articulationes carpometa-
    carpales
  articulationes carpometa-
    carpeae

ar·tic·u·la·tio *(continued)*
    a. carpometacarpalis pollicis
    a. carpometacarpea pollicis
    articulationes cartilagineae
    articulationes cinguli membri inferioris
    articulationes cinguli membri superioris
    a. cochlearis
    a. composita
    a. condylaris
    a. condylaris inversa
    articulationes costochondrales
    a. costotransversaria
    articulationes costovertebrales
    a. cotylica
    a. coxae
    a. crurotalaris
    a. cubiti
    a. cuneocuboidea
    a. cuneonavicularis
    a. ellipsoidea
    articulationes fibrosae
    a. genus
    a. humeri
    a. humeroradialis
    a. humero-ulnaris
    articulationes intercarpales
    articulationes intercarpeae
    articulationes interchondrales
    articulationes intercuneiformes
    articulationes intermetacarpales
    articulationes intermetacarpeae
    articulationes intermetatarsales
    articulationes intermetatarseae
    articulationes interphalangeae manus

ar·tic·u·la·tio *(continued)*
    articulationes interphalangeae pedis
    articulationes interphalangeales manus
    articulationes interphalangeales pedis
    articulationes intertarseae
    a. lumbosacralis
    articulationes manus
    a. mediocarpalis
    a. mediocarpea
    articulationes membri inferioris liberi
    articulationes membri superioris liberi
    articulationes metacarpophalangeae
    articulationes metacarpophalangeales
    articulationes metatarsophalangeae
    articulationes metatarsophalangeales
    a. ossis pisiformis
    a. ovoidalis
    articulationes pedis
    a. plana
    a. radiocarpalis
    a. radiocarpea
    a. radio-ulnaris
    a. radio-ulnaris distalis
    a. radio-ulnaris proximalis
    a. sacrococcygea
    a. sacroiliaca
    a. sellaris
    a. simplex
    a. sphaeroidea
    a. spheroidea
    a. sternoclavicularis
    articulationes sternocostales
    a. subtalaris
    articulationes synoviales
    a. talocalcanea
    a. talocalcaneonavicularis
    a. talocruralis
    a. talonavicularis

ar·tic·u·la·tio *(continued)*
  a. tarsi transversa
  articulationes tarsometa-
    tarsales
  articulationes tarsometa-
    tarseae
  articulationes thoracis
  a. tibiofibularis
  a. trochoidea
  articulationes vertebrales
  articulationes zygapophy-
    siales

ar·tic·u·la·tion
  acromioclavicular a.
  atlantoaxial a.
  atlantoaxial a., lateral
  atlantoaxial a., medial
  atlantodental a.
  atlantoepistrophic a.
  atlanto-occipital a.
  ball-and-socket a.
  bicondylar a.
  brachiocarpal a.
  brachioradial a.
  brachioulnar a.
  calcaneocuboid a.
  capitular a.
  carpal a's
  carpometacarpal a's
  carpometacarpal a., first
  carpometacarpal a. of
    thumb
  chondrosternal a's
  Chopart's a.
  composite a.
  compound a.
  condylar a.
  costocentral a.
  costosternal a's
  costotransverse a.
  costovertebral a's
  coxofemoral a. of Buisson
  craniovertebral a.
  crurotalar a.
  cubital a.
  cubitoradial a., inferior
  cubitoradial a., superior

ar·tic·u·la·tion *(continued)*
  cuneocuboid a.
  cuneonavicular a.
  a's of digits of foot
  a's of digits of hand
  a. of elbow
  ellipsoidal a.
  femoral a.
  fibrous a's
  gliding a.
  a's of hand
  a. of head of humerus
  a. of head of rib
  a. of hip
  humeroradial a.
  humeroulnar a.
  a. of humerus
  iliosacral a.
  intercarpal a's
  interchondral a's
  intercostal a's
  intercuneiform a's
  intermetacarpal a's
  intermetatarsal a's
  interphalangeal a's of fin-
    gers
  interphalangeal a's of foot
  interphalangeal a's of
    hand
  interphalangeal a's of toes
  intertarsal a's
  a. of knee
  lumbosacral a.
  mandibular a.
  maxillary a.
  a's of metacarpal bones
  metacarpocarpal a's
  metacarpophalangeal a's
  a's of metatarsal bones
  metatarsophalangeal a's
  neurocentral a.
  occipital a.
  occipito-atlantal a.
  ovoid a.
  petrooccipital a.
  phalangeal a's
  a. of pisiform bone
  pisocuneiform a.

ar·tic·u·la·tion *(continued)*
    pivot a.
    plane a.
    a. of pubis
    radiocarpal a.
    radioulnar a.
    radioulnar a., distal
    radioulnar a., inferior
    radioulnar a., proximal
    radioulnar a., superior
    sacrococcygeal a.
    sacroiliac a.
    saddle a.
    scapuloclavicular a.
    a. of shoulder
    simple a.
    spheroidal a.
    sternoclavicular a.
    sternocostal a's
    synovial a's
    talocalcaneonavicular a.
    talocrural a.
    talonavicular a.
    tarsometatarsal a's
    a's of thorax
    tibiofibular a's
    a's of toes
    transverse tarsal a.
    trochoidal a.
    uncovertebral a.
    a. of tubercle of rib
    zygapophyseal a's

ar·tic·u·la·ti·o·nes

ar·tic·u·lus *pl.* ar·tic·u·li

ar·ti·fact

ASA
    aspirin

ASD
    arthroscopic subacromial
      decompression

asep·tic
    a.-antiseptic

asys·tic

ASES
    American shoulder and el-
      bow system

Ash·hurst
    A. classification (for ankle
      fractures and sprains)
    A. sign

ASIF
    Association for the Study
      of Internal Fixation

ASIF clas·si·fi·ca·tion (for
  ankle fractures)

ASIS
    anterosuperior iliac spine

ASO (antistreptolysin O) ti·ter

as·par·tate ami·no·trans·fer·
  ase

as·par·tate trans·am·i·nase

as·phyx·ia

as·pi·ra·tion

as·pi·rin
    buffered a.
    a. and caffeine

as·say

as·sess·ment
    Frankel neurological a.
    functional capacity a.
    occupational therapy a.

as·sist
    first dorsal interosseous a.
    IP extension a.
    thumb interphalangeal ex-
      tension a.
    turnbuckle a.

as·sis·tant
    physical therapist a.

as·so·ci·a·tion
    aniridia–Wilms tumor a.
    CHARGE a.
    controlled a.
    MURCS a.
    VATER a.

AST
    aspartate transaminase

asta·sia

AST/GOT
    aspartate transami-
      nase:aspartate amino-
      transferase

as·the·nia

as·trag·a·lus
    aviator's a.

ASVG
    autologous saphenous vein
      graft

asym·met·ric

asym·me·try

asymp·to·mat·ic

asyn·er·gia

asy·no·via

At·a·sol

ata·vi·cus
    metatarsus a.

atax·ia
    Friedreich's a.
    locomotor a.

ate·los·teo·gen·e·sis

ATH (Anthropometric Total
  Hip) pros·the·sis

ath·er·o·ma

ath·ero·scle·ro·sis

ath·e·to·sis

At·lan·ta brace

at·lan·tad

at·lan·tal

at·lan·to·ax·i·al

at·lan·to·den·tal

at·lan·to·mas·toid

at·lan·to-oc·cip·i·tal

at·lan·to-odon·toid

at·las

at·lo·ax·oid

at·loi·do-oc·cip·i·tal

ato·nia

aton·ic

At·o·soy
    A. flap

ATP-glu·ta·thi·one

ATR
    angle of trunk rotation

atro·phia
    a. musculorum lipomatosa

at·ro·phied

at·ro·phy
    arthritic a.
    bone a.
    a. of disuse
    Erb's a.
    facioscapulohumeral mus-
      cular a.
    idiopathic muscular a.
    interstitial a.
    ischemic muscular a.
    juvenile muscular a.
    Landouzy-Dejerine a.
    leaping a.
    muscle a.
    muscular a.
    myopathic a.
    post-traumatic a. of bone
    pseudohypertrophic mus-
      cular a.
    rheumatic a.
    Sudeck's a.
    thigh a.
    Werdnig-Hoffmann spinal
      muscular a.

at·tach·ment
    Pearson's a.
    sternal a.

at·tack
    transient ischemic a. (TIA)

At·ten·bo·rough
   A. fully constrained device

at·ten·u·a·tion
   soft-tissue a.
   a. of tendons of hand

at·tri·tion
   a. of tendons of hand

atyp·i·cal

Au·franc
   A. concentric hip mold
   A. cup arthroplasty
   A.-Turner total hip re-
      placement

au·ran·o·fin

au·ro·ther·a·py

au·ro·thio·glu·cose

Aus·tin
   A. procedure

Aus·tin Moore
   A.M. arthroplasty
   A.M. hip prosthesis

au·to·am·pu·ta·tion

au·to·ci·ne·sis

au·tog·e·nous

au·to·graft
   bone-patellar
      tendon-bone a.
   free-revascularized a.

au·to·ki·ne·sis

au·to·ki·net·ic

avas·cu·lar

Aver·ill
   A. total hip replacement

AVF
   arteriovenous fistula

Avi·la
   A. approach to pelvis

Av·i·tene

AVM
   arteriovenous malforma-
      tion

AVN
   avascular necrosis

avul·sion

awl
   Kuntscher a.
   T-handled a.

ax·il·la *pl.* ax·il·lae

ax·is *pl.* ax·es
   central a.
   a. of cervical spine
   compromise a.
   femoral-tibial a.
   helical a. of motion
   instantaneous a. of rota-
      tion
   mechanical a.
   a. pelvis
   a. of pelvis
   a. of rotation
   tibiofemoral a.
   weight-bearing a.

ax·oid

ax·oi·de·an

ax·on

ax·on·ot·me·sis

Ayer·cil·lin

Azac·tam

aza·thio·prine

Az·lin

az·lo·cil·lin

Az·ma·cort

az·tre·o·nam

Azul·fi·dine

Baas·trup
  B's disease
  B's syndrome

Ba·bin·ski
  B. reflex
  B. sign
  B.-Fröhlich syndrome

ba·cil·lus *pl.* ba·cil·li
  acid-fast b. (AFB)

Ba·ciu
  B. and Filipiu arthrodesis

back
  flat b.
  functional b.
  hollow b.
  hump b.
  hunch b.
  poker b.
  saddle b.
  b. school

back·ache
  severe lumbar b.

back·bone

Back-Ese

Back·haus
  B. towel forceps

back·knee

Bac·trim

Badg·ley
  B. arthrodesis

Baer
  B's method

bag
  bean b.
  nuclear b.

Bag·by
  B. compression plate

Bah·ler
  Gschwend, Scheier, and B.
    elbow prosthesis

Bai·ley
  B. and Dubow osteotomy

Ba·ker
  B's cyst
  B. procedure
  B. tendon transfer
  B. and Hill osteotomy

Bal·four
  B. retractor

Bal·kan
  B. frame

ball
  chondrin b.

Bal·ler
  B.-Gerold syndrome

bal·lis·tics
  wound b.

Ba·lour·das
  Marcus, B., Heiple arthro-
    desis

Bal·ti·more Ther·a·peu·tic
  Work Sim·u·la·tor

Bam·ber·ger
  Marie-B. disease

band
  A b.
  brain b.
  calf b.
  contraction b.
  distal thigh b.
  H b.
  I b.
  iliotibial b.
  M b.
  Maissiat's b.
  Parham b.

band *(continued)*
    Partridge b.
    pelvic b.
    periosteal b.
    proximal thigh b.
    thigh b.
    Z b.
    zonular b.

ban·dage
    Ace b.
    Esmarch's b.
    Gibney b.
    Martin's b.
    Robert Jones b.

Ban·e·sin

Ban·kart
    B. lesion
    B. procedure
    B. repair
    B. tear

bank bone

Banks
    B. graft

bar
    abduction b.
    C b.
    calcaneocuboid b.
    calcaneonavicular b.
    congenital b.
    Denis Browne b.
    Fillauer b.
    lumbrical b.
    metatarsal b.
    opponens b.
    spreader b.
    talocalcaneal b.
    talonavicular b.
    tarsal b.
    torsion b.
    unsegmented b.
    Zielke sacral b.

Bard
    B.-Parker knife

Bar·den·ha·ben
    B's bone

Bar·det
    B.-Biedl syndrome

Bar·ker
    B's operation

Bar·kow
    B's ligament
    external ligaments of B.,
      plantar
    interosseous ligaments of
      B., internal

Barnes
    B's curve

baro·graph
    Elftman's b.

Barr
    B. procedure
    B.-Record procedure
    Ober-B. procedure

Bar·ré
    Guillain-B. syndrome

Bar·rett
    Bellemore and B. osteot-
      omy

Bar·ring·ton
    Dewar and B. procedure

Bar·sky
    B's operation

Bar·ton
    B's fracture
    B's operation

bas·i·lar

ba·sis *pl.* ba·ses
    b. metacarpalis
    b. metatarsalis
    b. ossis metacarpalis
    b. ossis metatarsalis
    b. ossis sacri
    b. patellae

ba·sis *(continued)*
  b. phalangis digitorum
    manus
  b. phalangis digitorum
    pedis
  b. scapulae

ba·si·ver·te·bral

ba·so·phil

basos
  basophils

Batch
  B. amputation

Batch·e·lor
  B.-Brown procedure

Bate·man
  B. arthroplasty
  B. bipolar prosthesis
  B. procedure
  B. prosthesis
  B. total hip replacement

bath
  contrast b.
  paraffin b.
  whirlpool b.

Bau·mann
  B. angle

BE
  below elbow

bead
  antibiotic b.

beak
  calcaneal b.

Beals
  B. auriculo-osteodysplasia
  B. syndrome

bean bag
  inflatable b.b.

bear·ing
  knee b.

Beath
  Harris-B. procedure
  Harrison-B. differential
    pressure mat

Beau·vais
  B. disease

Bech·tol
  B. prosthesis

Beck
  B's disease
  Kashin-B. disease

Beck·er
  B. tendon repair

Beck·man
  Adson-B. retractor
  B. retractor

Beck·with
  Adson-B. retractor

Bé·clard
  B's amputation

Bec·lo·vent

bed
  bone b.
  cancellous b.

bed·rest, bed rest

Bee·vor
  B. sign

be·hav·ior
  elastic b.
  plastic b.

Beh·çet
  B's syndrome

Bekh·te·rev
  B's disease
  B's spondylitis
  B. test
  Mendel-B. reflex

Bell
  B's palsy

Belle·more
    B. and Barrett osteotomy

Bel·li·ni
    B's ligament

belt
    control b.
    pelvic b.
    sacroiliac b.
    waist b.

bend·er
    driver-b.-extractor
    Rush b.

bend·ing

be·nign

Ben·nett
    B. basic hand splint
    B. dislocation
    B. fracture
    B. retractor

Bent·zon
    B's procedure

Ber·ger
    B's operation

Ber·man
    B. and Gartland procedure

Berndt
    B. hip ruler

Ber·tin
    B's ligament

Ber·to·lot·ti
    B's syndrome

Bes·nier
    B's rheumatism

Be·ta·dine
    B. dressing

Beth·a·prim

Bey·er
    B. rongeur

BFT
    bentonite flocculation test

B.H. Moore
    B.H.M. procedure

bi·ar·tic·u·lar

bi·car·bo·nate

bi·ceps
    b. brachii
    b. femoris

Bi·chat
    B's ligament

Bi·cil·lin

bi·cip·i·tal

Bick·el
    B. and Moe tendon trans-
      fer

bi·com·part·men·tal

bi·cor·ti·cate

Bie·brich
    B. scarlet–acid fuchsin so-
      lution

Biedl
    Bardet-B. syndrome

Bier
    B's amputation
    B's operation

bi·fur·ca·tion

Big·e·low
    B's ligament
    B. reverse maneuver
    B's septum

Bil
    bilirubin

bi·lat·er·al

bil·i·ru·bin
    total b.

bil·let

bind·er
    cloth b.

Bio·ce·ram

bio·ac·tive

bio·ce·ram·ic

bio·ce·ram·ics

bio·com·pat·i·bil·i·ty

bio·glass

bio·ma·te·ri·al

bio·me·chan·i·cal

bio·me·chan·ics

bio·met·al

Bio·met·ric pros·the·sis

Bio·met To·tal Toe pros·the·sis

bio·plant

bio·plas·tic

bi·op·sy
    bone marrow b.
    closed b.
    fine-needle aspiration b.
    needle b.
    open b.

bi·par·tite

bi·pen·ni·form

bi·po·lar

bi·por·tal

Bir·kett
    B's hernia

bis·acro·mi·al

Bish·op
    Luck-B. bone saw

bi·sil·i·ac

bit
    cannulated b.

bi·tro·chan·ter·ic

bi·valve
    Boston b.
    b. cervicis

Bix·ler
    Antley-B. syndrome

BK
    below knee

Black
    Staples-B.-Brostrom proce-
      dure

Black·burn
    B's calipers

Black·burne
    B. ratio
    B. and Peel index

blade
    locking b.
    trimmer b.

Blair
    B. arthrodesis
    B.-Brown skin graft

Blas·to·my·ces

Blauth
    B. knee prosthesis

Bla·zi·na
    Fox-B. procedure

Bleck
    B. procedure

block
    astragalocalcanean b.
    axillary b.
    bone b.
    calcaneus forefoot b.
    epidural b.
    femoral augmentation b.
    intercostal nerve b.
    interscalene nerve b.
    intravenous (IV) b.
    scalene b.
    spacer b.
    spinal b.
    surgical b.

block·age
    tendon b.

blood
    autologous b.
    complete b. count
    b. count
    red b. count
    white b. count

Bloom
    B. syndrome

Blount
    B. disease
    B. displacement osteotomy
    B. knee retractor
    B. osteotomy
    B. plate
    B. staple

blue
    aniline b.
    Evans b.

Blu·men·saat
    B. line

Blun·dell Jones
    B.J. hip osteotomy
    B.J. varus osteotomy

BMP
    bone marrow pressure

BMU
    basic multicellular unit

board
    spinal b.

body
    dense b's
    foreign b.
    infrapatellar fatty b.
    intravertebral b.
    loose b.
    melon-seed b.
    nemaline b's
    oryzoid b's
    rice b's
    Schmorl b.
    vertebral b.

Boeck
    B. sarcoid

Böh·ler
    B. angle
    B. splint
    B.-Braun frame
    B.-Braun splint

bol·lard

bolt
    distal locking b.
    expansion b.
    locking b.
    oblique locking b.
    proximal locking b.
    tibia b.
    tibial b.
    transverse locking b.
    Webb b.
    Zimmer tibia b.

bone
    AAA b.
    accessory b.
    accessory navicular b.
    acetabular b.
    acromial b.
    b. age
    Albers-Schönberg marble b's
    ankle b.
    astragaloid b.
    astragaloscaphoid b.
    back b.
    bank b.
    Bardeheben's b.
    b. bed
    breast b.
    Breschet's b.
    brittle b's
    calcaneal b.
    calf b.
    cancellated b.
    cancellous b.
    capitate b.
    carpal b's
    carpal b., central
    carpal b., first
    carpal b., fourth
    carpal b., great

bone *(continued)*
    carpal b., intermediate
    carpal b., radial
    carpal b., second
    carpal b., third
    carpal b., ulnar
    cartilage b.
    cavalry b.
    central b.
    chalk b.
    chalky b's
    coccygeal b.
    collar b.
    compact b.
    cortical b.
    corticocancellous b.
    costal b.
    cotyloid b.
    cribriform b.
    cuboid b.
    cuneiform b. of carpus
    cuneiform b., external
    cuneiform b., first
    cuneiform b., intermediate
    cuneiform b., internal
    cuneiform b., lateral
    cuneiform b., medial
    cuneiform b., middle
    cuneiform b., second
    cuneiform b., third
    b. curette
    decalcified b.
    demineralized b.
    b's of digits of foot
    b's of digits of hand
    b. disease
    b. dissection
    ectocuneiform b.
    endochondral b.
    entocuneiform b.
    episternal b.
    exercise b.
    femoral b.
    fibular b.
    b's of fingers
    flank b.
    freeze-dried b.
    fresh-frozen b.

bone *(continued)*
    funny b.
    hamate b.
    haunch b.
    healed b.
    b. healing
    heel b.
    hip b.
    b. hook
    humeral b.
    hyoid b.
    iliac b.
    innominate b.
    intermediate b.
    ischial b.
    b. island
    ivory b's
    Kiel b.
    Krause b.
    lamellar b.
    lenticular b. of hand
    lentiform b.
    b. liner
    long b.
    b. loss
    lunate b.
    marble b's
    b. mass
    mesocuneiform b.
    b. metabolism
    metacarpal b's
    metacarpal b., middle
    metacarpal b., third
    metatarsal b's
    mosaic b.
    multangular b., accessory
    multangular b., larger
    multangular b., smaller
    navicular b. of foot
    navicular b. of hand
    necrotic b.
    occipital b.
    odontoid b.
    osteonal b.
    osteoporotic b.
    pagetic b.
    pelvic b.
    perichondral b.

bone *(continued)*
    phalangeal b's of foot
    phalangeal b's of hand
    Pirie's b.
    pisiform b.
    postulnar b.
    primary b.
    primitive b.
    pubic b.
    pyramidal b.
    radial b.
    replacement b.
    resurrection b.
    reticulated b.
    retropulsed b.
    rider's b.
    sacral b.
    scaphoid b.
    scaphoid b. of foot
    scaphoid b. of hand
    scapular b.
    secondary b.
    secondary cuboid b.
    semilunar b.
    sesamoid b's
    sesamoid b's of foot
    sesamoid b's of hand
    shin b.
    short b.
    spoke b.
    spongy b.
    subchondral b.
    subperiosteal b.
    substitution b.
    suprasternal b's
    tarsal b's
    tarsal b., first
    tarsal b., second
    tarsal b., third
    thick b.
    thigh b.
    thoracic b's
    b's of toes
    trabecular b.
    trapezium b.
    trapezium b., lesser
    trapezium b. of Lyser
    trapezoid b.

bone *(continued)*
    trapezoid b. of Henle
    trapezoid b. of Lyser
    triangular b.
    triangular b. of tarsus
    triquetral b.
    tumor b.
    Type A, B, C b.
    ulnar b.
    ulnar carpal b.
    unciform b.
    uncinate b.
    ununited b.
    vesalian b.
    whettle b's
    wormian b's
    woven b.
    xiphoid b.

bone age
    TW_2 b.a.

bone bank

Bon·ner
    B's position

bony

boot
    cast b.

Bor·den
    B., Spencer, and Herndon
      osteotomy

bor·der
    b. of acetabulum
    external b.
    posterointernal b.
    sclerotic b.
    superior b.

Börje·son
    B.-Forssman-Lehmann
      syndrome

Bor·re·lia

bor·rel·i·o·sis
    Lyme b.

boss·ing
   carpal b.

Bos·ton
   B. bivalve
   B. brace
   B. orthosis

Bos·worth
   B. arthrodesis
   B. fracture
   B. lumbar spinal fusion
   B. procedure
   B. shelf procedure

Bot·ta
   B. prosthesis

bot·tom
   weavers' b.

Bou·chard
   B's nodes

Bou·in
   B's solution

Bour·gery
   B's ligament

bow
   traction b.

Bow·den
   B. single (dual, triple) con-
      trol cable

bow·ing
   anteromedial b.

bow·leg
   nonrachitic b.

bow·leg·ged

Bow·man
   B's disks

Boyd
   B's amputation
   B. graft
   B. stump
   B. and Anderson proce-
      dure

Boyd *(continued)*
   B. and Griffin classifica-
      tion (for trachanteric
      fractures of the femur)
   B. and McLeod procedure
   B. and Sisk procedure
   Bugg and B. procedure
   Speed and B. procedure

Boyes
   B. finger extension
   B. finger flexion
   B. thumb abduction
   B. wrist extension

brace
   Aircast b.
   Aircast walking b.
   Arnold b.
   Atlanta b.
   Bledsoe b.
   Blount b.
   Boston b.
   cast b.
   Charleston nighttime
      bending g.
   clam-shell b.
   dropfoot b.
   Fisher b.
   Florida b.
   49er knee b.
   Goldthwait b.
   Hudson b.
   hyperextension b.
   Jewett b.
   Jones b.
   Klenzak b.
   Knight-Taylor b.
   Kydex b.
   laminectomy b.
   Lenox Hill b.
   LSU reciprocation-gait or-
      thosis b.
   McKee b.
   Milwaukee b.
   Moe b.
   patellar cut-out b.
   Roylan tibia fracture b.
   SCOI shoulder b.

brace *(continued)*
    Seton hip b.
    SMo (stainless steel and
      molybdenum) b.
    SOMI b.
    Taylor b.
    Trinkle b.
    UBC (University of Brit-
      ish Columbia) b.
    walking b.
    Wilmington b.

bra·chia

bra·chi·al

bra·chio·cyl·lo·sis

bra·chio·cyr·to·sis

bra·chio·ra·di·a·lis

bra·chi·um *pl.* bra·chia

brachy·dac·ty·ly

brachy·sta·sis

brac·ing
    functional fracture b.

Brack·ett
    B. osteotomy

Brad·ford
    B. frame

Bra·gard
    B. sign

Brahms
    B. procedure

brain band

Brand
    B. finger flexion
    B. opponensplasty

Braun
    Böhler-B. frame
    Böhler-B. splint
    B. procedure
    B. skin graft

breast
    chicken b.
    funnel b.
    pigeon b.
    shoe-makers' b.

Brett
    B. arthrodesis
    B. osteotomy
    B. procedure
    B. and Campbell proce-
      dure

Breu·er·ton
    B. view

brev·i·col·lis

brev·i·flex·or

Brick·ner
    B. position

bridge
    anterior b.
    bony b.
    tarsal b.

Brig·ham
    B. unicompartmental ar-
      throplasty

brim
    quadrilateral b.

brise·ment
    b. forcé

Bris·saud
    B's scoliosis

Bris·tow
    B. procedure
    B.-Latarjet procedure

Brit·ish test

Brit·tain
    B. arthrodesis
    Dunn-B. arthrodesis
    Dunn-B. procedure
    Dunn-B. triple arthrodesis

broach

Bro·ca
   pilaster of B.

Brock·man
   B. procedure
   B.-Nissen arthrodesis

Bro·die
   B's abscess
   B's bursa
   B's disease
   B's knee
   B's ligament

Brog·greve
   B.-van Ness rotation oste-
      otomy

Bron·a·lide

Brook·er
   B.-Wills nail

Brooks
   B. technique
   B. and Saddon procedure

Bros·trom
   Staples-Black-B. procedure

Brown
   Batchelor-B. procedure
   Blair-B. skin graft
   B. procedure
   Matchett-B. hip prosthesis
   Matchett-B. total hip re-
      placement
   Radley, Liebig and B. ap-
      proach
   Radley, Liebig, and B. pro-
      cedure

Brown-Sé·quard
   B.-S. syndrome

Bruck
   B's disease

Brücke
   B's lines

Brud·zin·ski
   B. sign

Brun
   B. bone curette

Brunn
   Hassman, B., and Neer
      procedure

brush·ite

Bry·ant
   B's line
   B's sign
   B's traction

BTE
   Baltimore Therapeutic
      Equipment Work Simu-
      lator

Buch·holz
   B. unconstrained device
   St. George-B. ankle pros-
      thesis

Buch·oltz
   B. classification (for pelvic
      fractures)

Buck
   B's extension
   B's operation
   B. traction
   B.-Gramko pollicization

Bue·chel
   B.-Pappas total ankle re-
      placement

Buer·ger
   B's disease

buf·fer
   phosphate b.
   Trizma b.

Bugg
   B. and Boyd procedure
   Conrad-B. trapping

Buis·son
   coxofemoral articulation
      of B.

bulge
    disk b.

bump
    runner's b.

BUN
    blood urea nitrogen

bun·dle
    muscle b.
    neurovascular b.
    transverse b's of palmar
       aponeurosis
    Weissmann's b.

Bun·ge
    B's amputation

bun·ion
    tailor's b.

bun·ion·ec·to·my

bun·ion·ec·to·my

bun·ion·ette

Bun·nell
    B. finger flexion
    B. procedure
    B. pull out wire
    B. stitch
    B. suture
    B. tendon repair
    B. thumb adduction
    Stiles-B. finger flexion

bur
    diamond b.
    high-speed b.
    Midas Rex b.
    oval b.
    power b.

Bu·rem
    Flanagan and B. graft

Burk·hal·ter
    B. opponensplasty

Bur·meis·ter
    B. curve

Burns
    B. test

bur·sa pl. bur·sae
    b. of Achilles (tendon)
    acromial b.
    adventitious b.
    anconeal b.
    anconeal b. of triceps mus-
       cle
    b. anserina
    bicipital b.
    bicipitofibular b.
    bicipitoradial b.
    b. bicipitoradialis
    Brodie's b.
    calcaneal b.
    calcaneal b., subcutaneous
    b. of calcaneal tendon
    Calori's b.
    coracobrachial b.
    coracoid b.
    b. cubitalis interossea
    deep infrapatellar b.
    deltoid b.
    fibular b.
    b. of flexor carpi radialis
       muscle
    gastrocnemiosemimem-
       branous b.
    genual b., anterior
    genual b., external inferior
    genual bursae, internal
       superior
    genual b., posterior
    bursae glutaeofemorales
    gluteal b.
    gluteal intermuscular bur-
       sae
    gluteofascial bursae
    gluteofemoral bursae
    gluteotuberosal b.
    humeral b.
    iliac b., subtendinous
    b. iliaca subtendinea
    b. iliopectinea
    b. of iliopsoas muscle

bur·sa *(continued)*

inferior b. biceps femoris
muscle
infracondyloid b., external
infragenual b.
infrapatellar b.
infrapatellar b., deep
infrapatellar b., subcutaneous
infrapatellar b., superficial
inferior
b. infrapatellaris profunda
b. infrapatellaris subcutanea
intermediate b.
bursae intermusculares
musculorum gluteorum
interosseous cubital b.
intertubercular b.
b. intratendinea olecrani
ischiadic b.
b. ischiadica musculi glutei maximi
b. ischiadica musculi ob-
turatorii interni
ischial b. gluteus maximus
muscle
ischial b. internal obturator muscle
lateral b. gastrocnemius
muscle
b. of latissimus dorsi muscle
medial b. gastrocnemius
muscle
Monro's b.
b. mucosa
b. mucosa submuscularis
mucous b.
multilocular b.
b. musculi bicipitis femoris
inferior
b. musculi bicipitis femoris
superior
b. musculi coracobrachialis
b. musculi extensoris carpi
radialis brevis

bur·sa *(continued)*

b. musculi gastrocnemii
lateralis
b. musculi gastrocnemii
medialis
b. musculi infraspinati
b. musculi latissimi dorsi
b. musculi obturatoris interni
b. musculi piriformis
b. musculi poplitei
b. musculi sartorii propria
b. musculi semimembra-
nosi
b. musculi subscapularis
b. musculi teretis majoris
b. of olecranon
patellar b., deep
patellar b., middle
patellar b., prespinous
patellar b., subcutaneous
peroneal b., common
b. of piriform muscle
popliteal b.
b. of popliteal muscle
postcalcaneal b.
postcalcaneal b., deep
postgenual b., external
b. praepatellaris subcutanea
b. praepatellaris subfascialis
b. praepatellaris subtendinea
prepatellar b.
prepatellar b., middle
prepatellar b., subcuta-
neous
prepatellar b., subfascial
prepatellar b., subtendi-
nous
bursae prepatellares
b. prepatellaris profunda
b. prepatellaris subapo-
neurotica
pretibial b.
bursae propriae musculi
sartorii

bur·sa *(continued)*

    pyriform b.

    b. of quadratus femoris muscle

    radial b. of palm

    retrocondyloid b.

    retroepicondyloid b., lateral, deep

    sciatic b. gluteus maximus muscle

    sciatic b. obturator internus muscle

    b. sciatica musculi glutei maximi

    b. sciatica musculi obturatorii interni

    semimembranosogastrocnemial b.

    semimembranous b.

    semitendinous b.

    subachilleal b.

    subacromial b.

    b. subacromialis

    subcalcaneal b.

    subclavian b.

    subcoracoid b.

    subcrural b.

    b. subcutanea

    b. subcutanea acromialis

    b. subcutanea calcanea

    b. subcutanea infrapatellaris

    b. subcutanea malleoli lateralis

    b. subcutanea malleoli medialis

    b. subcutanea olecrani

    b. subcutanea prepatellaris

    b. subcutanea tuberositatis tibiae

    subcutaneous b.

    subcutaneous acromial b.

    subcutaneous b. lateral malleolus

    subcutaneous b. medial

    subcutaneous b. of olecranon

bur·sa *(continued)*

    subcutaneous synovial b.

    subcutaneous b. of tuberosity of tibia

    subdeltoid b.

    b. subdeltoidea

    subfascial b.

    subfascial synovial b.

    b. subfascialis

    b. subfascialis prepatellaris

    subiliac b.

    subligamentous b.

    submuscular b.

    submuscular synovial b.

    b. submuscularis

    subpatellar b.

    b. subtendinea

    b. subtendinea iliaca

    b. subtendinea musculi bicipitis femoris inferior

    b. subtendinea musculi gastrocnemii lateralis

    b. subtendinea musculi gastrocnemii medialis

    b. subtendinea musculi infraspinati

    b. subtendinea musculi latissimi dorsi

    b. subtendinea musculi obturatorii

    bursae subtendineae musculi sartorii

    b. subtendinea musculi subscapularis

    b. subtendinea musculi teretis majoris

    b. subtendinea musculi tibialis anterioris

    b. subtendinea musculi tibialis posterioris

    b. subtendinea musculi trapezii

    b. subtendinea musculi tricipitis brachii

    b. subtendinea prepatellaris

    subtendinous b.

bur·sa *(continued)*
- subtendinous b., medial
- subtendinous b. of anterior tibial muscle
- subtendinous b. of biceps femoris muscle, inferior
- subtendinous b. of infraspinatus muscle
- subtendinous b. of internal obturator muscle
- subtendinous b. of lateral head of gastrocnemius muscle
- subtendinous b. of obturator internus muscle
- subtendinous b. of posterior tibial muscle
- subtendinous bursae of sartorius muscle
- subtendinous b. of subscapularis muscle
- subtendinous synovial b.
- subtendinous b. of teres major muscle
- superficial infrapatellar b.
- superficial b. of knee
- superficial b. of olecranon
- superior b. of biceps femoris muscle
- supernumerary b.
- supra-anconeal b., intratendinous
- supracondyloid b., internal
- supracondyloid b., medial
- supragenual b.
- suprapatellar b.
- b. suprapatellaris
- synovial b.
- synovial b. of trochlea
- b. synovialis
- b. synovialis subcutanea
- b. synovialis subfascialis
- b. synovialis submuscularis
- b. synovialis subtendinea
- b. tendinis Achillis
- b. tendinis calcanei
- b. of tendon of Achilles

bur·sa *(continued)*
- trochanteric b., subcutaneous
- trochanteric b. gluteus maximus muscle
- trochanteric bursae of gluteus medius muscle
- trochanteric b. gluteus minimus muscle
- b. trochanterica musculi glutei maximi
- bursae trochantericae musculi glutei medii
- b. trochanterica musculi glutei minimi
- b. trochanterica subcutanea
- trochlear synovial b., trochlear
- tuberoischiadic b.
- ulnar b.
- ulnoradial b.
- vesicular b., ileopubic

bur·sae

bur·sal

bur·sal·o·gy

bur·sec·to·my

bur·si·tis
- Achilles b.
- adhesive b.
- calcific b.
- ischiogluteal b.
- olecranon b.
- patellar b.
- popliteal b.
- prepatellar b.
- radiohumeral b.
- retrocalcaneal b.
- scapulohumeral b.
- subacromial b.
- subdeltoid b.
- superficial calcaneal b.

bur·so·cen·te·sis

bur·so·lith

bur·sop·a·thy

bur·sos·co·py
    subacromial b.

bur·sot·o·my

Bur·stein
    Insall-B. II modular knee
        system
    Insall-B. prosthesis
    Wilson-B. total hip re-
        placement

Bus·quet
    B's disease

Bu·ta·tab

Bu·ta·zone

Butch·er
    B's saw

but·ton
    Richards b.

C
    cervical vertebrae (C1–C7)

CA
    cervicoaxial

Ca
    carpal
    carpal amputation

ca·ble
    Bowden single (dual, tri-
        ple) control c.
    control c.
    titanium c.

ca·chex·ia

ca·dence

café au lait spots

Caf·fe·drine

caf·feine
    acetaminophen and c.
    aspirin and c.

Caf·fey
    C's disease

cage
    elastic knee c.
    Swedish knee c.
    thoracic c.

Ca·lan·dri·el·lo
    C. hip reduction

Cal·an·druc·cio
    C. external fixator
    C. fixation device
    C. nail
    C. pressure apparatus
    C. total hip replacement
    C. triangular compression
        device

cal·ca·ne·al

cal·ca·ne·an

cal·ca·ne·itis

cal·ca·neo·apoph·y·si·tis

cal·ca·neo·as·trag·a·loid

cal·ca·neo·ca·vus

cal·ca·neo·cu·boid

cal·ca·ne·odyn·ia

cal·ca·neo·fib·u·lar

cal·ca·neo·na·vic·u·lar

cal·ca·neo·plan·tar

cal·ca·neo·scaph·oid

cal·ca·neo·tib·i·al

cal·ca·neo·val·go·ca·vus

cal·ca·ne·us *pl.* cal·ca·nei

cal·ca·no·dyn·ia

cal·car
    c. femorale
    c. pedis

cal·cif·e·di·ol

cal·cif·ic

cal·ci·fi·ca·tion
    metastatic c.
    periarticular c.

cal·ci·fied

cal·ci·fy

Cal·ci·mar

cal·ci·no·sis
    c. circumscripta
    c. intervertebralis
    tumoral c.

cal·cio·ki·ne·sis

cal·cio·ki·net·ic

Cal·ci·tite hip or·tho·sis

cal·ci·to·nin
  c.-salmon

cal·ci·tri·ol

cal·ci·um
  c. fluoride
  c. phospholipid phosphate
  c. pyrophosphate
  c. pyrophosphate dihydrate
  serum c.

cal·cu·lus *pl.* cal·cu·li
  articular c.
  joint c.

Cal·da·ni
  C's ligament

Cal·der·ol

Cald·well
  C. and Durham procedure
  C. and Durham tendon
    transfer

calf

cal·i·pers
  Blackburn's c.
  Cone's c.
  Gardner Wells c.
  skull c.
  Townley femur c.

Cal·la·han
  C. spondylotomy

Cal·lan·der
  C's amputation

Cal·la·way
  C's test

cal·los·i·tas

cal·los·i·ty

cal·lous

cal·lus
  bony c.
  central c.
  definitive c.
  ensheathing c.

cal·lus *(continued)*
  external c.
  inner c.
  intermediate c.
  internal c.
  medullary c.
  myelogenous c.
  permanent c.
  provisional c.
  Simpson c.
  temporary c.

Cal·nan
  C.-Nicole prosthesis

Ca·lo·ri
  C's bursa

Cal·vé
  C's disease
  C.-Perthes disease
  Legg-C.-Perthes disease

calx

Cam
  C. walker

cam·bi·um

cam·era *pl.* cam·eras, cam·erae
  gamma c.

Ca·mille
  Roy-C. plate

Camp·bell
  Brett and C. procedure
  C. arthrodesis
  C. graft
  C's ligament
  C. procedure
  C. and Akbarnia procedure
  C. tibial osteotomy
  modified C. arthrodesis

cam·po·spasm

camp·to·cor·mia

camp·to·cor·my

camp·to·dac·tyl·ia

camp·to·dac·tyl·ism

camp·to·dac·ty·ly

camp·to·me·lia

camp·to·me·lic

camp·to·spasm

Cam·u·ra·ti
   C.-Engelmann disease

ca·nal
   adductor c.
   calciferous c's
   carpal c.
   c's of cartilage
   central c. of modiolus
   crural c.
   crural c. of Henle
   femoral c.
   fibro-osseous c.
   flexor c.
   ganglionic c.
   Guyon's c.
   haversian c.
   hemal c.
   Hunter's c.
   iliac c.
   intersacral c's
   medullary c.
   neural c.
   nutrient c. of bone
   obturator c.
   obturator c. of pubic bone
   plasmatic c.
   sacral c.
   spinal c.
   subsartorial c.
   tarsal c.
   trefoil-shaped spinal c.
   triangular spinal c.
   vertebral c.
   Volkmann's c's

can·a·lic·u·li·za·tion

can·a·lic·u·lus *pl.* can·a·lic·u·li
   bone canaliculi
   haversian c.

ca·na·lis *pl.* ca·na·les
   c. adductorius
   c. carpalis
   c. carpi
   c. femoralis
   c. obturatorius
   c. sacralis
   c. spinalis
   c. subsartorialis
   c. vertebralis

can·cel·lous

can·cel·lus *pl.* can·cel·li

cane
   quad c.

can·na
   c. major
   c. minor

can·nu·la
   access c.
   Balgrist PN c.
   Concept arthroscopic c.

cap
   cartilaginous c.
   knee c.

ca·pac·i·tor

cap·e·line

Ca·pel·lo
   IMP-C. slimline abduction
     pillow
   C. total hip replacement

cap·il·lary

cap·i·tal

cap·i·tate

cap·i·ta·tum

cap·i·tel·lar

cap·i·tel·lum

cap·i·to·ham·ate

ca·pit·u·lar

ca·pit·u·lum *pl.* ca·pit·u·la
    c. costae
    c. fibulae
    c. humeri
    c. radii
    c. ulnae

cap·su·la *pl.* cap·su·lae
    c. articularis
    c. articularis acromioclavi-
      cularis
    c. articularis articulationis
      tarsi transversae
    c. articularis articula-
      tionum vertebrarum
    c. articularis atlantoaxi-
      alis lateralis
    capsulae articulares atlan-
      toepistrophicae
    c. articularis atlantooccipi-
      talis
    c. articularis calcaneocu-
      boidea
    c. articularis capitis costae
    capsulae articulares capi-
      tuli costae
    capsulae articulares carpo-
      metacarpeae
    c. articularis carpometa-
      carpea pollicis
    c. articularis costotrans-
      versaria
    c. articularis coxae
    c. articularis cubiti
    capsulae articulares digi-
      torum manus
    capsulae articulares digi-
      torum pedis
    c. articularis genus
    c. articularis humeri
    capsulae articulares inter-
      metacarpeae
    capsulae articulares inter-
      metatarseae

cap·su·la *(continued)*
    capsulae articulares inter-
      phalangearum manus
    capsulae articulares inter-
      phalangearum pedis
    c. articularis manus
    capsulae articulares meta-
      carpophalangeae
    capsulae articulares meta-
      tarsophalangeae
    c. articularis ossis pisifor-
      mis
    c. articularis radioulnaris
      distalis
    c. articularis sternoclavi-
      cularis
    c. articularis sternocostalis
    c. articularis talocalcanea
    c. articularis talocruralis
    c. articularis talonavicu-
      laris
    capsulae articulares tarso-
      metatarseae
    c. articularis tibiofibularis

cap·su·lar

cap·sule
    c. of ankle joint
    articular c.
    articular c., fibrous
    cartilage c.
    joint c.
    c. of lower limb
    c. of radiocarpal joint
    c. of subtalar joint
    synovial c.

cap·su·lec·to·my

cap·su·li·tis
    adhesive c.

cap·su·lo·de·sis
    palmar c.

cap·su·lo·lig·a·men·tous

cap·su·lo·plas·ty

cap·su·lor·rha·phy
    staple c.

cap·su·lot·o·my

cap·ut *pl.* cap·i·ta
  c. breve musculi bicipitis brachii
  c. breve musculi bicipitis femoris
  c. costae
  c. distortum
  c. femoris
  c. fibulae
  c. humerale musculi flexoris carpi ulnaris
  c. humerale musculi flexoris digitorum sublimis
  c. humerale musculi pronatoris teretis
  c. humeralis
  c. humeri
  c. humero-ulnare musculi flexoris digitorum superficialis
  c. laterale musculi gastrocnemii
  c. laterale musculi tricipitis brachii
  c. longum musculi bicipitis brachii
  c. longum musculi bicipitis femoris
  c. longum musculi tricipitis brachii
  c. mediale musculi gastrocnemii
  c. mediale musculi tricipitis brachii
  c. metacarpalis
  c. metatarsalis
  c. musculi
  c. obliquum musculi adductoris hallucis
  c. obliquum musculi adductoris pollicis
  c. ossis metacarpalis
  c. ossis metatarsalis
  c. phalangis digitorum manus

cap·ut *(continued)*
  c. phalangis digitorum pedis
  c. planum
  c. radiale musculi flexoris digitorum superficialis
  c. radii
  c. rectum musculi recti femoris
  c. reflexum musculi recti femoris
  c. tali
  c. transversum musculi adductoris hallucis
  c. transversum musculi adductoris pollicis
  c. ulnae
  c. ulnare musculi flexoris carpi ulnaris
  c. ulnare musculi pronatoris teretis

Car·a·fate

car·bon
  c. fiber

Car·den
  C's amputation

car·ies
  central c.
  dry c.
  c. fungosa
  necrotic c.
  c. sicca
  spinal c.

car·i·o·gen·ic

car·io·ge·nic·i·ty

car·i·os·i·ty

ca·ri·ous

Carle·ton
  C's spots

C-arm

Carne
  C. amputation

car·pal

car·pa·le

car·pec·to·my
    proximal row c.

Car·pen·ter
    C. sequence
    C. syndrome

car·po·car·pal

car·po·meta·car·pal

car·po·pe·dal

car·po·pha·lan·ge·al

car·pop·to·sis

car·pus
    c. curvus

Car·roll
    C. arthrodesis
    C. bone-holding forceps
    C. procedure
    C. and Taber arthroplasty

Car·ter
    C.-Rowe view

car·ti·lage
    aortic c.
    arthrodial c.
    articular c.
    calcified c.
    cellular c.
    circumferential c.
    connecting c.
    costal c.
    costal c., interarticular
    diarthrodial c.
    elastic c.
    ensiform c.
    epiphyseal c.
    falciform c's
    floating c.
    hyaline c.
    interarticular c.
    interarticular c. of little
      head of rib
    interosseous c.

car·ti·lage *(continued)*
    intervertebral c's
    investing c.
    mucronate c.
    obducent c.
    ossifying c.
    parenchymatous c.
    permanent c.
    precursory c.
    pulmonary c.
    reticular c.
    semilunar c. of knee joint,
      external
    semilunar c. of knee joint,
      internal
    sigmoid c's
    slipping rib c.
    sternal c.
    stratified c.
    temporary c.
    triquetral c.
    triquetrous c.
    triradiate c.
    triticeal c.
    triticeous c.
    Weitbrecht's c.
    xiphoid c.
    Y c.
    yellow c.

car·ti·la·gin·i·fi·ca·tion

car·ti·la·gin·i·form

car·ti·lag·i·noid

car·ti·lag·i·nous

car·ti·la·go *pl.* car·ti·lag·i·
nes
    c. articularis
    c. ensiformis
    c. epiphysialis
    cartilagines falcatae
    c. triquetra

car·ti·la·go·trop·ic

C.A.S.H. or·tho·sis

cast
    airplane c.

cast *(continued)*
  arm cylinder c.
  banjo c.
  bivalve c.
  body c.
  broomstick c.
  corrective c.
  Cotrel c.
  cylinder c.
  Dehne c.
  EDF (elongation, derotation, flexion) c.
  extension body c.
  fiberglass c.
  figure 8 c.
  flexion body c.
  gauntlet c.
  gel c.
  halo c.
  hanging c.
  hanging arm c.
  immobilization c.
  long-arm c.
  long-leg c.
  long-leg walking c.
  lower limb c.
  patellar tendon weight-bearing c.
  Petrie spica c.
  Quengle c.
  scoliosis c.
  serial c.
  short-arm c.
  short-leg c.
  short-leg walking c.
  slipper c.
  spica c.
  sugar tong c.
  turnbuckle c.
  univalve c.
  upper limb c.
  walking c.
  well-leg c.

cast·ing
  plaster c.

cat·ag·mat·ic

CAT-CAM
  contoured adducted trochanteric-controlled alignment method

ca·thep·sin

cath·e·ter
  arthrectomy c.
  Frazier-tipped suction c.
  Robinson c.

cath·e·ter·iza·tion

cath·ode

cat·lin

CAT scan

Cat·ter·all
  C. hip score

cau·da *pl.* cau·dae

cau·dad

cau·dal

cau·sal·gia

cau·ter·iza·tion

cau·tery

Cave
  C. and Rowe procedure

cav·i·tas *pl.* cav·i·ta·tes
  c. articularis
  c. glenoidalis
  c. medullaris

cav·i·ty
  absorption c's
  articular c.
  cotyloid c.
  glenoid c.
  joint c.
  marrow c.
  medullary c.
  popliteal c.
  sigmoid c. of radius
  sigmoid c. of ulna, greater
  sigmoid c. of ulna, lesser

ca·vo·val·gus

ca·vus

CAWO
  closing abductory wedge
    osteotomy

C bar

CBC
  complete blood count

cbc
  complete blood count

CC
  colony count
  coracoclavicular
  cord compression

Ccr
  creatinine clearance

CDH
  congenital dislocation of
    hip
  congenital dysplasia of the
    hip
  congenitally dysplastic hip

CDI
  Cotrel-Dubousset instru-
    mentation

C-D (Cotrel-Dubousset) sys·
  tem

CE (center edge) an·gle

CEC
  cauda equina compression

Ce·clor

cef·a·clor

cef·a·drox·il

Cef·a·dyl

cef·a·man·dole

Cef·a·nex

ce·faz·o·lin

ce·fix·ime

Cef·i·zox

cef·met·a·zole

Cef·o·bid

ce·fon·i·cid

cef·o·per·a·zone

ce·for·a·nide

Cef·o·tan

cef·o·tax·ime

cef·o·te·tan

ce·fox·i·tin

cef·ta·zi·dime

Cef·tin

cef·ti·zox·ime so·di·um

cef·tri·a·xone

ce·fu·rox·ime

ce·lio·myo·si·tis

cell
  bone c.
  cartilage c's
  contractile fiber c's
  Gegenbaur's c.
  LE c.
  muscle c.
  osseous c.
  osteoprogenitor c's
  sarcogenic c's
  satellite c's
  skeletogenous c.
  synovial c's
  tendon c's

cel·lu·li·tis

ce·ment
  acrylic bone c.
  antibiotic-impregnated c.
  bone c.
  methylmethacrylate c.
  tobramycin-methacrylate
    c.

cen·ter
    dentary c.
    epiotic c.
    c. of gravity
    ossification c.
    ossification c., primary
    ossification c., secondary
    splenial c.

cen·trode

cen·troid

cen·tro-os·teo·scle·ro·sis

cen·tro·scle·ro·sis

cen·trum *pl.* cen·tra
    c. ossificationis
    c. ossificationis primarium
    c. ossificationis secundarium
    c. vertebrae

ceph·a·lad

ceph·a·lex·in

ce·phal·ic

ceph·a·lo·med·ul·la·ry

ceph·a·lo·thin

ceph·a·pi·rin

ceph·ra·dine

Ce·por·a·cin

Ce·por·ex

ce·ram·ic
    bioactive c.

Ce·ram·ic ac·e·tab·u·lar com·po·nent

cer·clage
    c. wiring

cer·e·bral pal·sy
    ataxic c.p.
    athetoid c.p.
    diplegic c.p.
    flaccid c.p.
    spastic c.p.

cer·e·bro·vas·cu·lar

cer·vi·cal

cer·vi·co·cra·ni·al

cer·vi·co·cra·ni·um

cer·vi·co·dyn·ia

cer·vi·co·me·dul·la·ry

cer·vi·co·tho·rac·ic

cer·vi·co·tho·ra·co·lum·bo·sa·cral

C.E.S.

Chad·dock
    C. reflex
    C. sign

chain
    nuclear c.

Cham·ber·lain
    C's line

Chand·ler
    C. arthrodesis
    C. elevator
    C. procedure
    C. reamer
    C. retractor
    C. tendon transfer

Chang
    C. device

change
    Fairbanks c's

Cha·put
    C. tubercle

Char·cot
    C's disease
    C's foot
    C's joint
    C's syndrome
    Marie-C.-Tooth disease

CHARGE as·so·ci·a·tion

Charles·ton night·time bend·ing brace

char·ley horse

Charn·ley
C. arthrodesis
C. classification
C. hip arthroplasty
C. score
C. unconstrained device
C. unicompartmental device
C. zone
C. and Henderson arthrodesis
C.-Müller total hip replacement
DeLee and C. method

Chase
Albright and C. arthroplasty

Chas·sai·gnac
C's axillary muscle
C's tubercle

Chaves
C.-Rapp procedure

CHD to·tal hip re·place·ment

chei·lec·to·my

chei·ra·gra

cheir·ar·thri·tis

chei·ro·meg·a·ly

chei·ro·po·dal·gia

chei·ro·spasm

Che·kof·sky
Lewis and C. procedure

che·mo·nu·cle·ol·y·sis

Che·ney
Hajdu-C. syndrome

Cher·a·gan W/TMP

chest
alar c.
barrel c.
cobbler's c.

chest *(continued)*
flat c.
foveated c.
funnel c.
keeled c.
paralytic c.
phthinoid c.
pigeon c.
pterygoid c.
tetrahedron c.

Ches·ter
C's disease

Chi·a·ri
Arnold-C. syndrome
C. osteotomy
C. shelf procedure

chi·asm
c. of digits of hand
tendinous c. of flexor digitorum sublimis muscle

chi·as·ma *pl.* chi·as·ma·ta
c. tendinum digitorum manus

Chi·ene
C. test

chil·blain

CHILD syn·drome

Chilles
C. squeeze test

chip
bone c's

chi·ro·meg·a·ly

chi·ro·po·dal·gia

chi·ro·spasm

chis·el
cartilage c.
Meyerding c.
Smillie cartilage c.

chlor·am·phen·i·col

chlo·ride

chlo·ro·ma

Chlo·ro·my·ce·tin

chlor·o·quine

Cho
    C. procedure

Chol
    cholesterol

chol
    cholesterol

cho·les·ter·ol

cho·line
    c. and magnesium salicy-
       lates
    c. salicylate

Chol·me·ley
    Elmslie-C. procedure

chon·dral

chon·dral·gia

chon·dral·lo·pla·sia

chon·drec·to·my

chon·dric

chon·dri·fi·ca·tion

chon·dri·tis
    costal c.
    c. intervertebralis calca-
       nea

chon·dro·blast

chon·dro·blas·tic

chon·dro·blas·to·ma

chon·dro·cal·cin

chon·dro·cal·ci·no·sis

chon·dro·clast

chon·dro·cos·tal

chon·dro·cyte
    isogenous c's

chon·dro·dyn·ia

chon·dro·dys·pla·sia
    hereditary deforming c.
    metaphyseal c.
    metaphyseal c., Jansen
       type
    metaphyseal c., McKusick
       type
    metaphyseal c., Schmid
       type
    c. punctata
    c. punctata, Conradi-Hü-
       nermann type

chon·dro·dys·tro·phia
    c. calcificans congenita
    c. congenita punctata
    c. fetalis calcificans

chon·dro·dys·tro·phy
    familial c.
    hereditary deforming c.
    hyperplastic c.
    hypoplastic c.
    hypoplastic fetal c.
    c. malacia

chon·dro·epi·phys·e·al

chon·dro·epi·phys·itis

chon·dro·fi·bro·ma

chon·dro·gen·e·sis

chon·dro·gen·ic

chon·drog·ra·phy

chon·droid

chon·dro·it·ic

chon·dro·i·tin sul·fate

chon·dro·li·po·ma

chon·drol·o·gy

chon·drol·y·sis

chon·dro·ma
    joint c.
    synovial c.

chon·dro·ma·la·cia
    c. patellae

chon·dro·ma·to·sis
  Henderson-Jones c.
  synovial c.

chon·dro·ma·tous

chon·dro·meta·pla·sia
  synovial c.
  tenosynovial c.

chon·dro·mu·cin

chon·dro·mu·coid

chon·dro·mu·co·pro·tein

chon·dro·my·o·ma

chon·dro·myxo·fi·bro·ma

chon·dro·myx·o·ma

chon·dro·myxo·sar·co·ma

chon·dro·ne·cro·sis

chon·dro-os·se·ous

chon·dro-os·teo·dys·tro·phy

chon·dro·path·ia
  c. tuberosa

chon·dro·pa·thol·o·gy

chon·drop·a·thy
  patellar c.

chon·dro·phyte

chon·dro·pla·sia
  c. punctata
  c. punctata, Conradi-Hü-
    nermann type

chon·dro·plast

chon·dro·plas·tic

chon·dro·plas·ty

chon·dro·po·ro·sis

chon·dro·sar·co·ma
  clear cell c.
  dedifferentiated c.
  extraskeletal myxoid c.
  mesenchymal c.
  parosteal c.

chon·dro·sar·co·ma·to·sis

chon·dro·sis

chon·dro·skel·e·ton

chon·dros·te·o·ma

chon·dro·ster·nal

chon·dro·ster·no·plas·ty

chon·dro·tome

chon·drot·o·my

chon·dro·troph·ic

chon·dro·xi·phoid

cho·ne·chon·dro·ster·non

Cho·part
  C's amputation
  C's articulation
  C. dislocation
  C's joint
  C's operation

chor·da *pl.* chor·dae
  c. magna
  c. obliqua membranae in-
    terosseae antebrachii

chor·do·ma

cho·rea

Chot·zen
  Saethre-C. syndrome

Chris·man
  C. and Snook procedure

Chris·tian
  Hand-Schüller-C. disease

Chris·tian·sen
  C. arthroplasty
  C. total hip replacement

chrome
  cobalt c.

chro·mi·um

chryso·pho·re·sis

chryso·ther·a·py

chuck
    hand c.
    Jacobs c.
    T-handled c.
    universal c.

Chui·nard
    C. arthrodesis
    C. and Petersen arthro-
        desis
    modified C. arthrodesis

Chvos·tek
    C. sign
    C. test
    C.-Weiss sign
    Schultze-C. sign

Chy·mo·di·ac·tin

chy·mo·pa·pa·in

Ci·ba·cal·cin

cic·a·trix *pl.* cic·a·tri·ces

Ci·do·my·cin

ci·la·sta·tin
    imipenem and c.

ci·met·i·dine

cine·mat·iza·tion

cine·plas·tics

cin·e·plas·ty

cine·roent·geno·gram

cin·es·al·gia
    c. membri inferioris
    c. membri superioris
    c. pectorale
    c. pelvicum

Cin·tor semi·con·strained
    de·vice

Cip·ro

cip·ro·flox·a·cin

cir·ca·di·an

cir·cu·la·tion
    collateral c.

cir·cum·ar·tic·u·lar

cir·cum·fer·ence
    articular c.

cir·cum·fer·en·tia
    c. articularis
    c. articularis capitis ulnae
    c. articularis capituli ul-
        nae
    c. articularis radii

cis·tern
    terminal c's

CK
    creatine kinase

Cla·fo·ran

clamp
    Adair breast c.
    Allis c.
    Coker c.
    Halifax interlaminar c.
    Harrington hook c.
    hook c.
    interlaminar c.
    Kelly c.
    Köcher c.
    Lambert-Lowman bone c.
    Lewin bone holding c.
    Lowman bone c.
    Lowman bone c., modified
    Mayo c.
    meniscus c.
    mosquito c.
    patellar c.
    towel c.

Clan·cy
    C. procedure

Clarke
    C's column
    Osmond-C. procedure

clas·si·fi·ca·tion
    Aitken's c. (of epiphyseal
        fractures)

clas·si·fi·ca·tion *(continued)*
   Anderson and D'Alonzo c.
     (of odontoid fractures)
   Ashhurst c. (for ankle
     fractures and sprains)
   ASIF c. (for ankle frac-
     tures)
   Boyd and Griffin c. (for
     trochanteric fractures of
     the femur)
   Charnley c.
   Eaton c. (for trapeziometa-
     carpal joint degenera-
     tion)
   Epstein c. (for anterior
     dislocations of the hip)
   Epstein c. (for fractures
     associated with hip dislo-
     cation)
   Evans c. (for intratrochan-
     teric femoral fractures)
   Ficat c. (for avascular ne-
     crosis)
   Fielding c. (for subtro-
     chanteric fractures of the
     femur)
   Frankel c.
   Gustuilo c. (for open frac-
     tures)
   Harrington's c.
   Herbert's c. (for scaphoid
     fractures)
   Lauge-Hansen c. (for an-
     kle fracture)
   Marcus c. (for avascular
     necrosis of femoral head)
   Mason's c. (for radial head
     fractures)
   Neer c. (for fractures of
     the proximal humerus)
   Neer c. (for rotator cuff
     disease)
   Orthopaedic Trauma Asso-
     ciation c. (for tibial frac-
     ture stability)
   Portenoy's c.
   Rodichok's c.
   Salter-Harris c.

clas·si·fi·ca·tion *(continued)*
   Sukul c. (for scaphoid non-
     union)
   Winquist c. (for comminu-
     tion in femoral fracture)
   Winquist-Hansen c. (for
     comminution of femoral
     fractures)

clau·di·ca·tion
   jaw c.
   neurogenic c.
   vascular c.

Clau·sen
   Dyggve-Melchior-C. syn-
     drome

clav·i·cec·to·my

clav·i·cle

clav·i·cot·o·my

cla·vic·u·la

cla·vic·u·lar

cla·vic·u·lus *pl.* cla·vic·u·li

clav·i·pec·to·ral

clav·u·la·nate
   ticarcillin and c.

cla·vus *pl.* cla·vi
   c. mollis
   soft c.

claw·foot

claw·hand
   ulnar c.

Clee·man
   C's sign

clei·dag·ra

clei·dal

clei·dar·thri·tis

clei·do·cos·tal

clei·do·mas·toid

clei·sag·ra

Cle·land
    C. ligament

Cle·o·cin

C-Lex·in

click
    Ortolani's c.

clin·ar·thro·sis

clin·da·my·cin

cli·no·dac·tyl·ism

cli·no·dac·ty·ly

Clin·o·ril

clo·a·ca *pl.* clo·a·cae

clo·nus

Clo·quet
    C's fascia
    round ligament of C.
    septum of C.

clo·sure
    delayed primary c.
    primary c.
    secondary c.
    vest-over-pants c.

Clou·tier
    C. unconstrained device

Clow·ard
    C. graft
    C. impactor
    C. instrumentation
    C. method
    C. osteophyte elevator
    C. procedure
    C. self-retaining retractor

club·foot

club·hand
    radial c.
    ulnar c.

clunk
    patellar c.

Clut·ton
    C's joint

CMC
    carpometacarpal

cne·mi·al

cne·mis

cne·mi·tis

cne·mo·sco·li·o·sis

CO
    certified orthotist
    cervical orthosis

co·ag·u·la·tor
    Malis bipolar c.

co·a·li·tion
    calcaneocuboid c.
    calcaneonavicular c.
    cubonavicular c.
    naviculocuneiform c.
    talocalcaneal c.
    talonavicular c.
    tarsal c.

co·ar·tic·u·la·tion

co·balt
    c. chrome

Cobb
    C. angle
    C. elevator
    C. gouge
    C. method
    C.-Lippman technique

coc·cy·al·gia

coc·cy·dyn·ia

coc·cy·gal·gia

coc·cyg·e·al

coc·cy·gec·to·my

coc·cy·ge·rec·tor

coc·cyg·e·us

coc·cy·go·dyn·ia

coc·cy·got·o·my

coc·cy·odyn·ia

coc·cyx

Cock·ayne
    C's syndrome

Co·di·vil·la
    C. procedure
    C. V-Y advancement

Cod·man
    C. angle
    C's exercise
    C. pendulum exercises
    C. sign
    C's triangle
    C's tumor

co·ef·fi·cient
    stiffness c.

Cof·fin
    C.-Lowry syndrome
    C.-Siris syndrome

Co·hen
    C. syndrome

Cohn·heim
    C's areas
    C's fields

Co·ker
    C. clamp

col·chi·cine

Col·clough
    C. laminectomy rongeur

Cole
    C. osteotomy
    C. procedure

Cole·man
    C. procedure

col·la

col·la·gen
    microcrystalline c.
    woven bovine c.

col·la·gen·ase

col·la·ge·na·tion

col·la·gen·ic

col·lag·e·ni·tis

col·lag·e·no·blast

col·lag·e·no·cyte

col·la·gen·o·gen·ic

col·la·gen·o·sis

col·lag·e·nous

col·lapse
    carpal c.
    c. deformity
    scapholunate advanced c.
    subchondral c.

col·lar
    cervical c.
    hard c.
    Mayo-Thomas c.
    molded Thomas c.
    periosteal bone c.
    Plastazote c.
    soft c.
    Stifneck c.
    Thomas c.
    wire frame c.

col·lec·tion
    fluid c.

Col·les
    Ace-C. fixation device
    C's fracture
    C's ligament
    C. reverse fracture

Col·lins
    Mayo-C. retractor

col·lo·di·a·phys·e·al

col·loid·oph·a·gy

col·lum *pl.* col·la
    c. anatomicum humeri
    c. chirurgicum humeri
    c. costae
    c. distortum
    c. fibulae
    c. ossis femoris
    c. radii
    c. scapulae
    c. tali
    c. valgum

Co·lon·na
    C's operation
    C. shelf procedure

col·umn
    Clarke's c.
    dorsal c.
    dorsal c. of spinal cord
    dorsal lateral c. of spinal
      cord
    c. of Kölliker
    muscle c.
    spinal c.
    vertebral c.

co·lum·na *pl.* co·lum·nae
    c. vertebralis

com·a·tose

com·mi·nut·ed

com·mi·nu·tion

Com·mit·tee on Pros·thet·ic-
  Or·thot·ic Ed·u·ca·tion

com·mu·ni·ca·tion
    functional c.

Co·mol·li
    C's sign

com·pa·ges
    c. thoracis

com·part·ment
    anterior c.
    deep muscle c. of lower
      limb
    extensor c.

com·part·ment *(continued)*
    extensor tendon c.
    muscle c.
    muscle c. of lower limb
    muscular c.
    posterior muscle c. of
      lower limb

Com·part·men·tal II knee
  pros·the·sis

Com·pere
    C. and Wilson fusion
    Vulpius and C. procedure

com·plex
    capsuloligamentous c.
    jumped process c.
    major histocompatibility c.
      (MHC)
    triangular fibrocartilage c.

com·po·nent
    acetabular c.
    AML femoral c.
    ankle and foot prosthetic
      c.
    bipolar acetabular c.
    cell c.
    Ceramic acetabular c.
    condylar c.
    custom c.
    external knee c.
    femoral c.
    glenoid c.
    hemispheric press fit ace-
      tabular c.
    Judet femoral head c.
    metacarpal c.
    MHP (Mallory-Head pros-
      thesis) acetabular c.
    Omnifit-HA femoral c.
    PCA acetabular c.
    phalangeal c.
    radial c.
    single femoral c. with in-
      tramedullary stem
    stabilizer c.
    straight stem femoral c.
    talar c.

com·po·nent *(continued)*
    threaded acetabular c.
    tibial c.
    Trilock femoral c.
    T-Tap acetabular c.

Comp·quick CH₅₀

com·pres·sion
    cauda equina c.
    cord c.
    epidural spinal cord c.
    extradural c.
    iliac c.
    intermittent c.
    c. of nerve root
    root c.
    spinal cord c.
    vertical c.
    wedge c.

Con·ax·i·al an·kle pros·the·sis

con·cave

con·cen·trate
    platelet c's

Con·cept ar·thro·scop·ic can·nu·la

con·chio·lin·os·teo·my·eli·tis

con·cre·tion
    calculous c.
    tophic c.

con·di·tion·ing
    work c.

con·dy·lar

con·dy·lar·thro·sis

con·dyle
    extensor c. of humerus
    external c. of femur
    external c. of humerus
    external c. of tibia
    femoral c.
    fibular c. of femur
    flexor c. of humerus

con·dyle *(continued)*
    c. of humerus
    internal c. of femur
    internal c. of humerus
    internal c. of tibia
    lateral c. of femur
    lateral c. of humerus
    lateral c. of tibia
    medial c. of femur
    medial c. of humerus
    medial c. of tibia
    occipital c.
    radial c. of humerus
    c. of scapula
    tibial c. of femur
    ulnar c. of humerus

con·dy·lec·to·my
    DuVries plantar c.

con·dyl·i·cus

con·dy·lot·o·my

con·dy·lus *pl.* con·dy·li
    c. humeri
    c. lateralis femoris
    c. lateralis humeri
    c. lateralis tibiae
    c. medialis femoris
    c. medialis humeri
    c. medialis tibiae
    c. occipitalis
    c. tibialis femoris

Cone
    C's calipers

con·fig·u·ra·tion
    fracture c.

con·gen·i·tal

con·gru·en·cy

con·gru·ent

Con·ju·gat·ed Es·tro·gens C.S.D.

con·nec·tion
    intertendinous c.

con·nec·ti·vi·tis
  systemic c.

con·nec·tor
  pedicle c.

con·nex·us *pl.* con·nex·us
  c. intertendineus

Co·noi·dal an·kle pros·the·
  sis

Con·rad
  C.-Bugg trapping

Con·radi
  chondrodysplasia punc-
    tata, C.-Hünermann type
  C's disease
  C's syndrome

Con·ray

con·struct
  D-L c.

con·trac·tion
  carpopedal c.
  concentric c.
  Dupuytren's c.
  eccentric c.
  isokinetic c.
  palmar c.
  tetanic c.
  tonic c.

con·trac·ture
  Dupuytren's c.
  flexion c.
  flexion c. of knee
  ischemic c.
  ischemic muscle c.
  muscle c.
  organic c.
  organic muscle c.
  postpoliomyelitic c.
  postpoliomyelitic muscle c.
  Volkmann's c.

con·tra·lat·er·al

con·tre·coup

con·trol
  myoelectric c.
  nudge c.
  rotary c.

con·tu·sion

co·nus *pl.* co·ni
  c. medullaris

con·va·les·cence

con·vex

con·vex·i·ty
  left c.
  right c.

con·vexo·ba·sia

con·vul·sion

con·vul·sive

cook·ie
  shoe c.

Coon·rad
  C. elbow prosthesis

Coo·per·nail
  C. sign

co·os·si·fi·ca·tion

co·os·si·fy

Cope·land
  C. and Howard procedure

copo·dys·ki·ne·sia

co·poly·mer
  polyactide-glycolide c.

cor·a·co·acro·mi·al

cor·a·co·bra·chi·al·is

cor·a·co·cla·vic·u·lar

cor·a·co·hu·mer·al

cor·a·coid

cor·a·coi·di·tis

cor·a·co·ra·di·a·lis

cor·a·co·ul·nar·is

cord
    heel c.
    oblique c. of elbow joint
    spinal c.
    Weitbrecht's c.

cor·do·ma

cor·dot·o·my

corn
    hard c.
    soft c.

cor·nu *pl.* cor·nua
    c. coccygeale
    c. coccygeum
    c. inferius marginis falci-
      formis
    sacral c.
    c. sacrale
    c. superius marginis falci-
      formis

cor·pec·to·my
    anterior c.

cor·pus *pl.* cor·po·ra
    c. adiposum infrapatellare
    c. calcanei
    c. claviculae
    c. costae
    c. fibulae
    c. humeri
    c. metacarpalis
    corpora oryzoidea
    c. ossis femoris
    c. ossis ilii
    c. ossis ischii
    c. ossis metacarpalis
    c. ossis metatarsalis
    c. ossis pubis
    c. phalangis digitorum
      manus
    c. phalangis digitorum
      pedis
    c. radii
    c. sterni
    c. tali
    c. tibiae
    c. ulnae

cor·pus *(continued)*
    c. vertebrae
    c. vertebrale

cor·pus·cle
    bone c.
    cartilage c.
    Golgi's c's
    tendon c's

cor·set
    dorsal lumbar c.
    lumbosacral c.
    surgical c.

cor·tex *pl.* cor·ti·ces

cor·ti·co·can·cel·lous

cor·ti·co·car·ti·lag·i·nous

cor·ti·cot·o·my

cor·ti·co·tro·pin

Cor·tro·phin-Zinc

cos·me·sis

cos·ta *pl.* cos·tae
    c. cervicalis
    c. fluctuans
    costae fluitantes
    c. prima
    costae spuriae
    costae verae

cos·tae

cos·tal

cos·tal·gia

cos·ta·lis

cos·ta·tec·to·my

cos·tec·to·my

cos·ti·car·ti·lage

cos·ti·cer·vi·cal

cos·tif·er·ous

cos·ti·form

cos·ti·spi·nal

cos·to·cen·tral

cos·to·cer·vi·ca·lis

cos·to·chon·dral

cos·to·cla·vic·u·lar

cos·to·cor·a·coid

cos·to·gen·ic

cos·to·in·fe·ri·or

cos·to·scap·u·lar

cos·to·scap·u·lar·is

cos·to·ster·nal

cos·to·ster·no·plas·ty

cos·to·su·pe·ri·or

cos·to·tome

cos·tot·o·my

cos·to·trans·verse

cos·to·trans·ver·sec·to·my

cos·to·ver·te·bral

cos·to·xiph·oid

Co·trel
    C. cast
    C. traction
    C.-Dubousset instrumenta-
       tion

Co·trim

Cot·ter·ill
    Osborne and C. procedure

cot·ting

Cot·ton
    C. tibial osteotomy

cot·ton·oid

Cot·trell
    Lucas and C. osteotomy

cot·y·lo·pu·bic

cot·y·lo·sa·cral

Couch
    C., DeRosa, and Throop
       procedure

count
    colony c.
    complete blood c.
    red blood c.
    reticulocyte c.
    white blood c.

coun·ter
    extended c.

coun·ter·ex·ten·sion

coun·ter·trac·tion
    c. de fouet

coup·ling
    capacitive c.

cov·er
    soft cosmetic c.

Cow·per
    C's ligament
    pubic ligament of C.

coxa
    c. adducta
    c. brevis
    c. flexa
    c. magna
    c. plana
    c. saltans
    c. valga
    c. vara
    c. vara luxans

cox·al·gia

cox·ar·thria

cox·ar·thri·tis

cox·ar·throc·a·ce

cox·ar·throp·a·thy

cox·ar·thro·sis

cox·itis
    c. fugax
    senile c.

cox·odyn·ia

coxo·fem·o·ral

cox·ot·o·my

coxo·tu·ber·cu·lo·sis

CP
    cerebral palsy
    certified prosthetist

CPK
    creatine phosphokinase

CPK Ag·a·ro-Stain

CPM
    continuous passive motion

CPOE
    Committee on Prosthetic-
    Orthotic Education

CPPD
    calcium pyrophosphate di-
    hydrate
    calcium pyrophosphate di-
    hydrate disease

Cr
    creatinine

Craig
    Kramer, C., and Noel oste-
    otomy

Cra·mer
    C's splint

cramp
    accessory c.
    foot c.
    muscle c.

cra·ni·ad

cra·ter·iza·tion

Craw·ford
    C.-Adams cup arthroplasty
    C.-Adams dexterity test

crawl

C-re·ac·tive pro·tein

crease
    skin c.

cre·a·tine ki·nase

cre·at·i·nine

creep

Cre·go
    C. hip reduction
    C. osteotomy

crep·i·tant

crep·i·ta·tion

crep·i·tus
    articular c.
    bony c.
    false c.
    joint c.
    silken c.

cres·cent
    articular c.

crest
    anterior c. of fibula
    anterior c. of tibia
    deltoid c.
    femoral c.
    gluteal c.
    c. of greater tubercle of
        humerus
    c. of hypotrochanteric
        fossa
    iliac c.
    iliopectineal c. of iliac
        bone
    iliopectineal c. of pelvis
    iliopectineal c. of pubis
    c. of ilium
    interosseous c. of fibula
    interosseous c. of radius
    interosseous c. of tibia
    interosseous c. of ulna
    intertrochanteric c.
    intertrochanteric c., ante-
        rior
    c. of larger tubercle
    lateral c. of fibula

crest *(continued)*
    c. of lesser tubercle
    c. of little head of rib
    medial c. of fibula
    c. of neck of rib
    obturator c. (anterior)
    pectineal c. of femur
    pubic c.
    c. of pubis
    radial c.
    rough c. of femur
    sacral c.
    sacral c., articular
    sacral c., external
    sacral c., intermediate
    sacral c., lateral
    sacral c., medial
    c. of smaller tubercle
    spinal c. of Rauber
    c. of spinous processes of
     sacrum
    supinator c.
    c. of supinator muscle
    supracondylar c. of hu-
     merus, lateral
    supracondylar c. of hu-
     merus, medial
    tibial c.
    ulnar c.

CREST syn·drome

cris·ta *pl.* cris·tae
    c. anterior fibulae
    c. anterior tibiae
    c. capitis costae
    c. colli costae
    c. femoris
    c. iliaca
    c. interossea fibulae
    c. interossea radii
    c. interossea tibiae
    c. interossea ulnae
    c. intertrochanterica
    c. lateralis fibulae
    c. medialis fibulae
    c. musculi supinatoris
    c. obturatoria
    c. pubica

cris·ta *(continued)*
    cristae sacrales articulares
    c. sacralis intermedia
    c. sacralis lateralis
    c. sacralis media
    c. sacralis mediana
    c. supracondylaris lateralis
     humeri
    c. supracondylaris medi-
     alis humeri
    c. tuberculi majoris
    c. tuberculi minoris
    c. ulnae

cri·te·ri·on *pl.* cri·te·ria
    McNab criteria
    New York criteria
    Rome criteria

CRITOE
    capitellum, radial head,
     internal condyle, troch-
     lea, olecranon, external
     condyle (ossification se-
     quence in elbow)

cross-bridges

cross·foot

cross-link·ing

cross·union

Crou·zon
    C. syndrome

CRP
    C-reactive protein

cru·re·us

crus *pl.* cru·ra
    medial c. of external in-
     guinal ring

crutch

Crutch·field
    C. tongs

Cru·veil·hier
    adipose ligament of knee
     of C.

Cru·veil·hier *(continued)*
  anterior pubic ligament of
    C.
  C's joint
  C's ligaments
  glenoid ligaments of C.
  interosseous ligament of
    C., costovertebral
  interosseous ligament of
    C., transversocostal

cry·mo·dyn·ia

cryo·pre·cip·i·tate

crypt
  synovial c.

crys·tal
  calcium pyrophosphate c.
  calcium pyrophosphate di-
    hydrate (CPPD) c's
  hydroxyapatite c.
  monosodium urate c.
  sodium urate c.

Crys·ta·pen

Crys·ti·cil·lin

C&S
  culture & sensitivity

CSF
  cerebrospinal fluid

C-spine
  cervical spine

CSR
  corrected sedimentation
    rate

CT/dis·kog·ra·phy

CTLSO
  cervicothoracolumbosacral
    orthosis

Cub·bins
  C. procedure

cu·bi·to·car·pal

cu·bi·to·ra·di·al

cu·bi·tus
  c. valgus
  c. varus

cu·boid

cu·cul·la·ris

cuff
  condylar c.
  musculotendinous c.
  rotator c.

cul·ture
  anaerobic c.
  c. of CSF
  c. and sensitivity
  special c.

cu·ne·i·form

cu·neo·cu·boid

cu·neo·na·vic·u·lar

cu·neo·scaph·oid

cup
  acetabular c.
  arthroplasty c.
  Arthropor I acetabular c.
  Arthropor II acetabular c.
  Duraloc acetabular c.
  Gripper Plus acetabular c.
  Laing concentric hip c.
  c. loosening
  Omnifit acetabular c.
  SuperCup acetabular c.

cup po·si·tion·er

Cup·ri·mine

cu·ret

cu·ret·tage
  trephine c.

cu·rette
  angled c.
  bone c.
  Brun bone c.
  Epstein reverse-angle c.
  long c.
  Ring c.

cu·rette *(continued)*
  short c.
  straight c.

cur·rent
  interferential c.

Cur·tis
  C. arthroplasty

cur·va·ture
  cylindrical c.
  degree of c.
  Pott's c.
  spinal c.
  trochlear c.

curve
  Barnes' c.
  Burmeister c.
  compensated c.
  concave c.
  convex c.
  flattening of normal lum-
    bar c.
  Herzog's c.
  load deformation c.
  lumbar c.
  spinolaminar c.
  tension c's
  thoracic c.
  thoracolumbar c.

cur·vi·lin·e·ar

Cush·ing
  C's disease

cu·ti·cle

cut·ter
  cushion throat wire c.
  dowel c.
  multiple action c.
  pin c.
  wire c.

C-wash·er

cy·a·no·sis

cy·a·not·ic

Cy·bex dy·na·mom·e·ter

cyc·lar·thro·di·al

cyc·lar·thro·sis

cy·cle
  gait c.

cy·clo·phos·pha·mide

cyl·in·der
  Leydig's c's

cyl·in·drar·thro·sis

cyl·lo·sis

Cyr·i·ax
  C's syndrome

cyr·to·sis

cyst
  aneurysmal bone c.
  Baker's c.
  bone c.
  bursal c.
  ganglion c.
  ganglionic c.
  inclusion c.
  mucous c.
  popliteal c.
  sacral c.
  simple bone c.
  solitary bone c.
  subchondral c.
  subsynovial c.
  synovial c.
  thecal c.
  unicameral bone c.

cy·tom·e·try
  flow c.

Cy·to·tec

Cy·tox·an

Czer·ny
  C's disease
  C's suture

D
distal
dorsal vertebrae (D1–D12)

D/3
distal third

DA
degenerative arthritis

Da·cron

dac·ty·lo·camp·so·dyn·ia

dac·ty·lo·gry·po·sis

dac·ty·lol·y·sis

dac·ty·lo·meg·a·ly

dac·ty·lo·spasm

dac·ty·lus

D'Alon·zo
Anderson and D'A. classi-
fication (of odontoid fractures)

dal·ton

Da·na
D. total shoulder

Dan·los
Ehlers-D. syndrome

Dar·rach
D. procedure
D.-Hughston-Milch frac-
ture

Das Gup·ta
D. G. procedure

Da·tril

D'Au·bigne
D'A. hip prosthesis
D'A. procedure

Da·vid
D's disease

Da·vid *(continued)*
D. skin graft

Da·vis
D. arthrodesis

Daw·barn
D. sign

Day
Riley-D. syndrome

DCP
dynamic compression plate

Deane
D. unconstrained device

de·ar·tic·u·la·tion

De·beyre
D. procedure

dé·bride·ment

de·bulk·ing

de·cal·ci·fi·ca·tion

de·cal·ci·fy

Dec·lo·my·cin

de·com·pres·sion
anterior d.
canal d.
core d.
direct d.
indirect d.
joint d.
late anterior d.
posterolateral d.
d. of spinal cord
subacromial d.
transpedicular d.

de·cor·ti·ca·tion

Dee
D. elbow prosthesis

65

de·fect
  bone d.
  cervical vertebral d.
  cold d.
  cortical d.
  cortical fibrous d.
  fibrous cortical d.
  filling d.
  metaphyseal fibrous d.
  neural-tube d.
  subcortical d.
  subperiosteal cortical d.

def·er·ves·cence

de·fi·cien·cy
  congenital limb d.
  fibular d.
  intercalary longitudinal
    limb d.
  intercalary transverse
    limb d.
  proximal femoral focal d.
  proximal focal femoral d.
  terminal longitudinal
    limb d.

def·i·cit
  neurologic d.

de·form·i·ty
  arthritic d.
  boutonnière d.
  buttonhole d.
  collapse d.
  congenital d.
  equinovarus d.
  fixed d.
  flexion d.
  fracture d.
  gun stock d.
  Haglund's d.
  hatchet head d.
  Ilfeld-Holder d.
  intrinsic minus d.
  intrinsic plus d.
  Kirner d.
  kyphotic d.
  lateral spine d.
  lobster-claw d.

de·form·i·ty *(continued)*
  Madelung's d.
  Nalebuff d. (Types I-V)
  progressive d.
  recurvatum d.
  rocker-bottom d.
  rotary d.
  seal-fin d.
  shepherd's crook d.
  silver fork d.
  Sprengel's d.
  swan-neck d.
  thumb-in-palm d.
  ulnar drift d.
  varus d.
  Velpeau's d.
  Volkmann's d.

de·gen·er·a·tion
  disk d.

de·gen·er·a·tive

de·gree
  d. of curvature

de·his·cence

Dehne
  D. cast

de·hy·dro·gen·ase

De·jer·ine
  Landouzy-D. dystrophy
  D. sign

De·la·di·ol

Del·ad·i·ol-40

de Lange
  de L. syndrome

De·Lee
  D. zone
  D. and Charnley method

Del·es·tro·gen

De·Lorme
  D. exercise

Del·rin

del·ta
    d. mesoscapulae

Del·ta·lin

del·toid

del·toi·de·us

del·to·pec·to·ral

dem·e·clo·cy·cline
    d. hydrochloride

De·mia·noff
    D. sign

demi·fac·et
    inferior d. for head of rib
    superior d. for head of rib

de·min·er·al·iza·tion

de·min·er·al·ized

Den·ham
    D. fixation device

Den·is Browne
    D.B. bar
    D.B. splint

dens *pl.* den·tes
    d. axis
    d. epistrophei

den·si·tom·e·try
    dual-photon d.
    photon d.

den·si·ty
    bone d.

den·ta·ta

De·nu·cé
    D's ligament

de·os·si·fi·ca·tion

De·Pal·ma
    D. prosthesis

De·pen

dep·Gyn·o·gen

De·po-Es·tra·di·ol

De·po·gen

de·pos·it

dep·o·si·tion
    calcium pyrophosphate di-
        hydrate d.

de·pres·sion
    congenital chondrosternal
        d.
    radial d.
    supratrochlear d.

de Quer·vain
    de Q's disease
    de Q's fracture

de·range·ment
    Hey's internal d.
    internal d. of joint

Der·by
    D. nail

de·riv·a·tive
    purified protein d.

der·ma·to·ar·thri·tis
    lipid d.
    lipoid d.

der·ma·to·ma

der·ma·tome

der·ma·tom·ic

der·mod·e·sis

De·Ro·sa
    Couch, D., and Throop
        procedure

De·sault
    D. dislocation
    D. sign

des·mal·gia

des·mec·ta·sis

des·min

des·mi·tis

des·mo·cy·to·ma

des·mo·dyn·ia

des·mog·e·nous

des·mog·ra·phy

des·moid
   extraabdominal d.
   periosteal d.

des·mol·o·gy

des·mo·ma

des·mop·a·thy

des·mo·pla·sia

des·mo·plas·tic

des·mor·rhex·is

des·mo·sis

des·mot·o·my

Des·Prez
   Kiehn-Earle-D. procedure

des·truc·tion
   bone d.
   discovertebral d.
   geographic bone d.
   moth-eaten bone d.
   permeative bone d.

Deutsch·län·der
   D's disease

de·vi·a·tion
   radial d.
   ulnar d.

de·vice
   Ace-Colles fixation d.
   Ace-Fischer fixation d.
   Anametric unconstrained
      d.
   bilateral fixation d.
   Buchholz unconstrained d.
   Calandruccio fixation d.
   Calandruccio triangular
      compression d.
   Chang d.
   Charnley unconstrained d.

de·vice *(continued)*
   Charnley unicompartmen-
      tal d.
   Cintor semiconstrained d.
   circular fixation d.
   Cloutier unconstrained d.
   compression d.
   constrained elbow d.
   Cruciate Condylar uncon-
      strained d.
   Deane unconstrained d.
   Denham fixation d.
   Duocondylar uncon-
      strained d.
   Duopatellar unconstrained
      d.
   Eriksson unconstrained d.
   fixation d.
   four-bar fixation d.
   Fox internal fixation d.
   Freeman-Swanson uncon-
      strained d.
   Geomedic unconstrained d.
   Guepar fully constrained
      d.
   Gunston unconstrained d.
   Gunston-Hult unicompart-
      mental d.
   Gustuilo unconstrained d.
   Herbert fully constrained
      d.
   Herbert unconstrained d.
   Hoffman fixation d.
   Hoffman-Vital fixation d.
   HSS semiconstrained d.
   ICLH unconstrained d.
   Ikuta fixation d.
   Ilizarov fixation d.
   Insall/Burstein semicon-
      strained d.
   internal fixation d.
   Kaneda d.
   Kennedy ligament aug-
      mentation d.
   Kinematic fully con-
      strained d.
   Kinematic II semicon-
      strained d.

de·vice *(continued)*

    Lacey fully constrained d.
    LAI unconstrained d.
    ligament augmentation d.
    Liverpool unconstrained d.
    Lubinus unconstrained d.
    Lund unicompartmental d.
    MacIntosh unicompart-
      mental d.
    Marmor unconstrained d.
    Monticelli-Spinelli
      fixation d.
    Noiles fully constrained d.
    Norris humeral extraction
      d.
    Oxford unicompartmental
      d.
    PCA unconstrained d.
    PCA unicompartmental d.
    Polycentric unconstrained
      d.
    quadrilateral fixation d.
    RAM unconstrained d.
    Rezaian fixation d.
    Ring unconstrained d.
    RMC unconstrained d.
    Robert Brigham semicon-
      strained d.
    Roger Anderson fixation d.
    St. George fully con-
      strained d.
    St. George sledge unicom-
      partmental d.
    semicircular fixation d.
    semiconstrained d.
    semiconstrained elbow d.
    Sevastano unconstrained
      d.
    Sevastano unicompart-
      mental d.
    Sheehan fully constrained
      d.
    Shiers fully constrained d.
    SKI unconstrained d.
    Spherocentric fully con-
      strained d.
    Stabilocondylar semicon-
      strained d.

de·vice *(continued)*

    Stanmore fully con-
      strained d.
    Statak d.
    Sukhtian-Hughes
      fixation d.
    SureTac d.
    TCCK unconstrained d.
    terminal d. for upper limb
      prosthesis
    Total Condylar semicon-
      strained d.
    Townley unconstrained d.
    traction d.
    triangular fixation d.
    UCI unconstrained d.
    unconstrained elbow d.
    unilateral fixation d.
    unilateral unicompart-
      mental d.
    Vidal-Ardrey fixation d.
    Volkov-Oganesyan
      fixation d.
    Wagner fixation d.
    Walldius fully constrained
      d.
    Wasserstein fixation d.
    Waugh unconstrained d.
    Whiteside semiconstrained
      d.
    Wright unconstrained d.
    YIS unconstrained d.

De·war

    D. and Barrington proce-
      dure

Dex·i·tac

Dex·on

Dex·on su·ture

dex·ter

dex·tro·ro·to·sco·li·o·sis

D/3 frac·ture

di·a·be·tes

di·ac·e·tyl

di·ac·la·sis

Di·a·gen

di·ag·no·sis

di·a·gram
 bending moment d.
 butterfly d.
 stress-strain d.

di·a·phragm

di·aph·y·sary

di·aph·y·se·al

di·a·phys·ec·to·my

di·aph·y·si·al

di·aph·y·sis *pl.* di·aph·y·ses

di·aph·y·si·tis
 tuberculous d.

di·ap·la·sis

di·a·poph·y·sis

di·ar·thric

di·ar·thro·di·al

di·ar·thro·ses

di·ar·thro·sis *pl.* di·ar·thro·
 ses
 d. rotatoria

di·ar·tic·u·lar

di·as·ta·sic

di·as·ta·sis
 ankle mortise d.

di·a·stat·ic

di·a·stem·a·to·my·e·lia

di·as·to·le

di·a·stroph·ic

di·a·ther·my

di·ath·e·sis
 gouty d.

dia·tri·zo·ate
 d. meglumine

Di·a·tri·zo·ate-60

Dick·son
 D. osteotomy
 D.-Diveley procedure

di·clo·fe·nac

Di·dro·nel

Dief·fen·bach
 D's amputation

Die·ker
 Miller-D. syndrome

di·eth·yl·amine sal·i·cyl·ate

di·eth·yl·stil·bes·trol

dif·fer·ence
 rib vertebral angle d.
 T (translation) d.
 translation d.

dif·fuse

di·flu·ni·sal

dig·it
 supernumerary d.

dig·i·tal

dig·i·ta·tion

dig·i·to·plan·tar

dig·i·tus *pl.* dig·i·ti
 d. annularis
 d. hippocraticus
 d. malleus
 digiti manus
 d. medius
 d. minimus manus
 d. minimus pedis
 d. mortuus
 digiti pedis
 d. primus (I) manus
 d. primus (I) pedis
 d. quartus (IV) manus
 d. quartus (IV) pedis
 d. quintus (V) manus

dig·i·tus *(continued)*
    d. quintus (V) pedis
    d. secundus (II) manus
    d. secundus (II) pedis
    d. tertius (III) manus
    d. tertius (III) pedis
    d. valgus
    d. varus

di·hy·dro·tach·ys·te·rol

di·la·tor

Di·mon
    D. osteotomy
    D. and Hughston proce-
       dure

dim·ple
    d's of Venus

Di·o·val

DIP
    distal interphalangeal

di·phos·pho·nate

di·ple·gia

di·ple·gic

Di·sal·cid

dis·ar·tic·u·la·tion
    ankle d.
    elbow d.
    hip d.
    knee d.
    shoulder d.
    wrist d.

Dis·case

dis·cec·to·my

dis·ci·tis

dis·co·ge·net·ic

dis·co·gen·ic

dis·cog·ra·phy

dis·coid·ec·to·my

dis·cop·a·thy

dis·cop·a·thy *(continued)*
    traumatic d.

dis·co·ver·te·bral

dis·crim·i·na·tion
    two-point d.

dis·cus *pl.* dis·ci
    d. articularis
    d. articularis articulationis
       acromioclavicularis
    d. articularis articulationis
       radioulnaris distalis
    d. articularis articulationis
       sternoclavicularis
    d. interpubicus
    disci intervertebrales

dis·di·a·clast

dis·ease (see also under
  syndrome)
    Albers-Schönberg d.
    apatite deposition d.
    Apert's d.
    arterial occlusive d.
    Baastrup's d.
    back d.
    back and neck d.
    Bamberger-Marie d.
    Beauvais' d.
    Beck's d.
    Bekhterev's d.
    Blount d.
    bone d.
    bony d. of spine
    Brodie's d.
    Bruck's d.
    Buerger's d.
    Busquet's d.
    Caffey's d.
    caisson d.
    calcium hydroxyapatite
      deposition d.
    calcium pyrophosphate
      deposition d. (CPDD)
    calcium pyrophosphate di-
      hydrate d.
    Calvé-Perthes d.

dis·ease *(continued)*
- Camurati-Engelmann d.
- cartilage d.
- cervical disk d.
- Charcot's d.
- Charcot joint d.
- Charcot-Marie-Tooth d.
- Chester's d.
- collagen d.
- collagen vascular d.
- congenital back d.
- congenital d. of spine
- Conradi's d.
- coxa d.
- CPPD d.
- crystal deposition d's
- Cushing's d.
- Czerny's d.
- David's d.
- degenerative disk d. (Types I-III)
- degenerative joint d.
- de Quervain's d.
- Deutschländer's d.
- disk d.
- diver's d.
- Duchenne's d.
- Duchenne-Griesinger d.
- Duplay's d.
- Durante's d.
- Engelmann's d.
- Engel-Recklinghausen d.
- Erb's d.
- Erb-Goldflam d.
- Erb-Landouzy d.
- fibromuscular d.
- Fleischner's d.
- Forestier d.
- Freiberg's d.
- Garré's d.
- Gaucher's d.
- Gibney's d.
- Gorham's d.
- Haglund's d.
- Hagner's d.
- Hand-Schüller-Christian d.
- Heberden's d.

dis·ease *(continued)*
- Henderson-Jones d.
- hip-joint d.
- Hodgkin's d.
- Hoffa's d.
- infectious bone d.
- inflammatory joint d.
- Jaffe's d.
- Jaffe-Lichtenstein d.
- Jansen's d.
- joint d.
- juvenile Paget d.
- Kaschin-Beck d.
- Kashin-Beck d.
- Kawasaki d.
- Kienböck's d.
- Köhler's d.
- Köhler's bone d.
- Köhler's second d.
- Köhler-Pellegrini-Stieda d.
- König's d.
- Kümmell's d.
- Kümmell-Verneuil d.
- Kuskokwim d.
- Landouzy-Dejerine d.
- Larsen's d.
- Larsen-Johansson d.
- Legg's d.
- Legg-Calvé d.
- Legg-Calvé-Perthes d.
- Legg-Calvé-Waldenström d.
- Leriche's d.
- Letterer-Siwe d.
- lipid storage d.
- Lobstein's d.
- Lou Gehrig's d.
- lower motor neuron d.
- Luft's d.
- lumbar disk d.
- Lyme d.
- MacLean-Maxwell d.
- Madelung's d.
- Marie's d.
- Marie-Bamberger d.
- Marie-Charcot-Tooth d.
- Marie-Strümpell d.
- Martin's d.

dis·ease *(continued)*
  metabolic d.
  metabolic bone d.
  Meyer-Betz d.
  milk alkali d.
  Miller's d.
  Milroy's d.
  mixed connective tissue d.
  motor neuron d.
  Mozer's d.
  Münchmeyer's d.
  muscle d.
  musculoskeletal d.
  neck and back d.
  nerve root d. of spine
  neurologic d.
  Niemann-Pick d.
  occlusive arterial d.
  Ollier's d.
  Osgood-Schlatter d.
  Otto's d.
  Paas' d.
  Paget d.
  Panner's d.
  Parkinson's d.
  Pellegrini's d.
  Pellegrini-Stieda d.
  Perrin-Ferraton d.
  Perthes' d.
  plaster-of-Paris d.
  policeman's d.
  Poncet's d.
  Pott's d.
  Preiser's d.
  Pyle's d.
  Quervain's d.
  Raynaud's d.
  Recklinghausen's d. of
    bone
  rheumatoid d.
  Rust's d.
  sacroiliac d.
  Schanz's d.
  Scheuermann's d.
  Schlatter's d.
  Schlatter-Osgood d.
  Schmorl's d.
  Schwediauer's d.

dis·ease *(continued)*
  Sever's d.
  Sinding-Larsen-Johansson
    d.
  Stieda's d.
  Still's d.
  Strümpell-Marie d.
  Sudeck's d.
  Swediaur's (Schwediauer's)
    d.
  synovial d.
  Thiemann's d.
  Tietze's d.
  tissue d.
  Trevor's d.
  upper motor neuron d.
  Verneuil's d.
  Verse's d.
  vibration d.
  Volkmann's d.
  von Recklinghausen's d.
  Voorhoeve's d.
  Vrolik's d.
  Waldenström's d.
  Wartenberg's d.
  Wegner's d.
  Werdnig-Hoffmann d.
  Wilson's d.

DISH
  diffuse idiopathic skeletal
    hyperostosis

DISI
  dorsiflexed intercalated
    segment instability

dis·in·ser·tion

dis·joint

disk
  A d.
  Amici's d.
  anisotropic d.
  anisotropous d.
  articular d.
  Bowman's d's
  d. bulge
  contained d.

disk *(continued)*
    Engelmann's d.
    epiphyseal d.
    extruded d.
    growth d.
    Hensen's d.
    I d.
    interarticular d.
    intermediate d.
    interpubic d.
    intervertebral d's
    intra-articular d.
    isotropic d.
    J d.
    M d.
    noncontained d.
    protruded d.
    d. protrusion
    Q d.
    ruptured d.
    sequestered d.
    slipped d.
    thin d.
    transverse d.
    Z d.

dis·kec·to·my
    automated percutaneous
      lumbar d.
    laser d.
    limited surgical d.
    open d.
    percutaneous d.

dis·ki·tis
    infectious d.

dis·ko·gen·ic

dis·ko·gram

dis·kog·ra·phy
    computed tomographic
      (CT) d.
    midline lumbar d.
    posterior lumbar d.

dis·ko·scope

dis·lo·ca·tio
    d. erecta

dis·lo·ca·tion
    acromioclavicular d.
    d. of ankle
    Bell-Dally d.
    Bennett's d.
    central d. of hip
    Chopart d.
    closed d.
    complete d.
    complicated d.
    compound d.
    congenital d.
    congenital d. of hip
    congenital d. of knee
    consecutive d.
    Desault d.
    direct injury d.
    divergent d.
    elbow d.
    facet d.
    fracture d.
    fracture d. of hip
    frank d.
    habitual d.
    hand d.
    hip d.
    implant d.
    incomplete d.
    interphalangeal joint d.
    Kienböck's d.
    Lisfranc's d.
    lunate d.
    milkmaid's d.
    Monteggia's d.
    Nélaton's d.
    old d.
    open d.
    partial d.
    d. of patella
    pathologic d.
    perilunate d.
    posterior d.
    primitive d.
    proximal interphalangeal
      joint d.
    recent d.
    recurrent d.
    rotary d.

dis·lo·ca·tion *(continued)*
  shoulder d.
  simple d.
  Smith's d.
  spine d.
  spontaneous hyperemic d.
  subastragalar d.
  subcoracoid d.
  subglenoid d.
  subspinous d.
  tarsal d.
  transscaphoid perilunate d.
  traumatic d.
  wrist d.

dis·mem·ber·ment

dis·or·der
  arterial d.
  conversion d.
  myeloproliferative d.
  somatization d.
  venous d.

dis·place·ment
  angular d.
  axillary disk d.
  central disk d.
  classic disk d.
  disk d.
  double disk d.
  dual-level disk d.
  foraminal disk d.
  high lumbar disk d
  lateral disk d.
  load d.
  lumbar disk d.
  posterolateral disk d.

dis·sec·tion
  blunt d.
  bone d.
  sharp d.

dis·sec·tor
  elevator-d.
  Penfield d.
  Woodson d.

dis·tad

dis·tal

distal/3
  distal third

dis·tract

dis·trac·tion

dis·trac·tor
  AO/ASIF femoral d.
  femoral d.
  Harrington d.

di·var·i·ca·tion

Di·ve·ley
  Dickson-D. procedure

di·ver·tic·u·lum *pl.* di·ver·tic·u·la
  ganglion d.
  synovial d.

Do·bie
  D's globule
  D's layer
  D's line

Dodd's pills

Do·la·nex

Dol·ge·sic

Do·lo·bid

do·lor *pl.* do·lo·res
  d. coxae

dome
  superior d. of acetabulum

do·nor

Dop·pler
  bidirectional D.

dor·sa

dor·sad

dor·sal

dor·sal·gia

dor·sa·lis

dor·si·duct

dor·si·flex·ion

dor·si·flex·or

dor·si·spi·nal

dor·so·an·te·ri·or

dor·so·ceph·a·lad

dor·so·dyn·ia

dor·so·in·ter·cos·tal

dor·so·in·ter·os·se·al

dor·so·lat·er·al

dor·so·lum·bar

dor·so·me·di·al

dor·so·me·di·an

dor·so·nu·chal

dor·so·pos·te·ri·or

dor·so·ra·di·al

dor·so·sa·cral

dor·so·scap·u·lar

dor·sum *pl.* dor·sa
    d. of foot
    d. of hand
    d. manus
    d. pedis
    d. of scapula
    d. scapulae

Dor·yx

dose
    roentgen absorbed d.

dow·el
    postfibular d.

dow·el cut·ter
    Cloward d.c.

Down
    D. syndrome

Down·ing
    D. cartilage knife
    D. retractor

Doxy-Caps

Doxy·cin

doxy·cy·cline

Drag·stedt
    D. skin graft

drain·age
    dependent d.
    incision and d.

dress·ing
    adaptic d.
    Betadine d.
    compression d.
    dry d.
    figure 8 d.
    gauze d.
    high Dye d.
    iodoform d.
    Kerlix d.
    Kling d.
    Koch-Mason d.
    low Dye d.
    occlusive d.
    plaster of Paris d.
    pressure d.
    protective d.
    rigid d. for amputated part
    saline d.
    Shanz d.
    sterile d.
    Telfa d.
    universal hand d.
    Velpeau d.
    wet-to-dry d.
    Xeroform d.

drift
    lateral d.
    radial d.
    ulnar d.

drill
    air d.
    anticavitational d.
    cannulated d.
    hand d.
    high-speed d.

drill *(continued)*
   Midas Rex d.

drill·ing
   transcapular d.

Dris·dol

dri·ver
   Flatt d.
   Harrington hook d.
   Jewett d.
   Küntscher d.
   Massie d.
   prosthesis d.
   staple d.

driv·er-bend·er-ex·trac·tor
   Rush d.-b.-e.

driv·er-ex·trac·tor
   Hansen-Street d.-e.
   Ken d.-e.
   McReynolds d.-e.
   Schneider d.-e.
   Zimmer d.-e.

drop
   foot d.
   d. phalangette
   wrist d.

drop·foot

drop·sy
   articular d.

drug
   nonsteroidal anti-inflam-
      matory d.

Du·bi·net
   D. hip prosthesis

Du·bous·set
   Cotrel-D. instrumentation

Du·bow
   Bailey and D. osteotomy

Du·bo·witz
   D. syndrome

Du·chenne
   D's disease

Du·chenne *(continued)*
   D. muscular dystrophy
   D's type
   D. type muscular dystro-
      phy

duc·til·i·ty

Du·gas
   D. test

Du·hot
   D's line

dumb·bell
   d's of Schäfer

Dun·lop
   D. traction

Dunn
   D. procedure
   D.-Brittain arthrodesis
   D.-Brittain procedure
   D.-Brittain triple arthro-
      desis
   Weaver and D. procedure

Duo·con·dy·lar un·con·
strained de·vice

Duo·pa·tel·lar un·con·
strained de·vice

Du·play
   D's disease

du·pli·ca·tion
   Wassel thumb d.

Du·puy·tren
   D's amputation
   D's contraction
   D's contracture
   D's fracture
   D's operation
   D's sign

du·ra

Du·ra·cil·lin

Du·ra-Es·trin

Du·ra·gen

Du·ra·loc ac·e·tab·u·lar cup

Du·ran·te
    D's disease

du·ra·tion
    stride d.

Dur·ham
    Caldwell and D. procedure
    Caldwell and D. tendon
        transfer

Du·ri·cef

du·rot·o·my
    dorsal d.
    midline d.

Du·ver·nay
    Graber-D. procedure

Du·ver·ney
    D's fracture

Du·Vries
    D. plantar condylectomy
    D. procedure

dwarf
    ateliotic d.
    diastrophic d.
    micromelic d.
    phocomelic d.

dwarf·ism
    achondroplastic d.
    diastrophic d.
    exostotic d.
    pituitary d.
    polydystrophic d.

Dwy·er
    D. instrumentation
    D. osteotomy
    D. procedure
    D. spinal implant

Dygg·ve
    D.-Melchior-Clausen syn-
        drome

dy·na·mi·za·tion

dy·na·miz·ing

dy·na·mom·e·ter
    bulb d.
    Cybex d.
    Cybex II d.
    isokinetic d.
    Jamar d.
    Kin-Com d.

dys·ar·thro·sis

dys·chon·dro·pla·sia

dys·chon·dro·ste·o·sis
    Leri-Weill d.

dys·col·lag·e·no·sis

dys·equi·lib·ri·um
    postural d.

dys·es·the·sia

dys·func·tion
    desmogenous d.
    extensor mechanism d.

dys·gen·e·sis
    alar d.
    epiphyseal d.

dys·ki·ne·sia

dys·os·teo·gen·e·sis

dys·os·to·sis
    cleidocranial d.
    d. enchondralis epiphy-
        saria
    metaphyseal d.

dys·pla·sia
    acromesomelic d.
    arteriohepatic d.
    camptomelic d.
    chondroectodermal d.
    congenital d. of hip
    congenital hip d.
    cortical fibrous d.
    craniometaphyseal d.
    diaphyseal d.
    diastrophic d.
    epiarticular osteochondro-
        matous d.
    epiphyseal d.

dys·pla·sia *(continued)*
  epiphyseal d. multiplex
    congenita
  d. epiphysealis hemimelica
  d. epiphysealis multiplex
  d. epiphysealis punctata
  fibrous d.
  fibrous d. (of bone)
  fibrous d. ossificans pro-
    gressiva
  frontometaphyseal d.
  geleophysic d.
  intracortical fibrous d.
  Kniest d.
  Kozlowski spondylometa-
    physeal d.
  Langer mesomelic d.
  metaphyseal d.
  metatropic d.
  monostotic fibrous d.
  multiple epiphyseal d.
  Namaqualand hip d.
  osteofibrous d.
  polyostotic fibrous d.
  progressive diaphyseal d.
  pseudoachondroplastic
    spondyloepiphyseal d.
  Pyle metaphyseal d.
  spondyloepiphyseal d.
  spondyloepiphyseal d. con-
    genita
  spondyloepiphyseal d.
    tarda
  Streeter's d.
  thanatophoric d.

dys·pro·si·um

dys·ra·phism

dys·tro·phia
  d. brevicollis

dys·troph·in

dys·tro·phy
  Albright's d.
  Becker's d.
  Becker's muscular d.
  Dejerine-Landouzy d.
  distal d.
  distal muscular d.
  Duchenne type muscular
    d.
  Duchenne-Landouzy d.
  Erb's d.
  facioscapulohumeral d.
  facioscapulohumeral mus-
    cular d.
  Fröhlich's adiposogenital
    d.
  Gowers type muscular d.
  Jeune thoracic d.
  Landouzy's d.
  Landouzy-Dejerine d.
  Leyden-Möbius d.
  limb girdle d.
  limb-girdle muscular d.
  muscular d.
  myotonic d.
  ocular d.
  progressive muscular d.
  pseudohypertrophic d.
  pseudohypertrophic mus-
    cular d.
  reflex sympathetic d.
  Simmerlin's d.

Earle
  Kiehn-E.-DesPrez proce-
    dure

Ea·ton
  E. classification (for trape-
    ziometacarpal joint de-
    generation)
  E's implant arthroplasty
  E. prosthesis
  E. trapezium implant
  E.-Littler arthroplasty

Eb
  E. paralysis

ebo·na·tion

ebur·na·tion

ec·chy·mo·sis *pl.* ec·chy·mo·
ses

Eck·er
  E., Lotke, and Glazer ten-
    don transfer

ec·pinch

ec·ta·sia
  dural e.

ec·to·con·dyle

ec·to·cu·ne·i·form

ec·to·pec·to·ra·lis

ec·top·ic

ec·tos·te·al

ec·to·sto·sis

ec·tro·dac·tyl·ia

ec·tro·dac·ty·lism

ec·tro·dac·ty·ly

E-Cyp·i·o·nate

ED
  elbow disarticulation

ede·ma
  constrictive e.
  marrow e.
  rheumatismal e.

edem·a·tous

Eden
  E.-Hybbinette procedure
  E.-Lange procedure

EDF (elongation, derotation,
  flexion) cast

Ed·gar·ton
  E.-Grand thumb adduction

Ed·wards Mod·u·lar Spi·nal
Sys·tem

EEC syn·drome

ef·fect
  fetal alcohol e's
  fetal aminopterin e's
  fetal hydantoin e's
  fetal rubella e's
  fetal trimethadione e's
  fetal valproate e's
  fetal varicella e's
  fetal warfarin e's
  maternal PKU fetal e's
  rocker bottom e.

ef·fu·sion
  knee e.
  synovial e.

Ef·te·khar
  E. prosthesis

Eg·gers
  E. bone plate
  E. plate
  E. screw
  E. tendon transfer

Eh·lers
  E.-Danlos syndrome

Ei·cher
    E. hip prosthesis

elas·tic·i·ty
    modulus of e.

elas·to·fi·bro·ma

elas·to·mer
    HP-100 silicone e.
    silicone e.

el·bow
    baseball e.
    baseball pitchers' e.
    boxer's e.
    disarticulation of e.
    fused e.
    golfer's e.
    intraarticular fusion of e.
    javelin thrower's e.
    Little Leaguer's e.
    milkmaid's e.
    miners' e.
    nursemaids' e.
    pulled e.
    reverse tennis e.
    tennis e.
    thrower's e.

elec·tro·bi·ol·o·gy

elec·tro·cau·ter·iza·tion

elec·tro·cau·tery

elec·trode
    meniscectomy e.
    surface e.

Elec·tro·dy·no·graph

elec·tro·go·ni·om·e·ter

elec·tro·myo·gram

elec·tro·myo·graph

elec·tro·my·og·ra·phy

elec·tro·pho·re·sis
    hemoglobin e.
    serum protein e.

el·e·va·tor
    Adson periosteal e.
    Chandler e.
    chisel-edge e.
    Cloward osteophyte e.
    Cobb e.
    curve-tipped rib e.
    curved e.
    e.-dissector
    Harrington spinal e.
    Key e.
    Key periosteal e.
    Lagenbach e.
    Langenbeck periosteal e.
    Liberator e.
    osteophyte e.
    Penfield e.
    periosteal e.
    periosteum e.
    proximal femoral e.
    rib e.
    Rotator Cuff Liberator e.
    spinal e.
    straight e.
    Woodson e.

el·e·va·tor-dis·sec·tor
    Freer e.-d.

Elft·man
    E's barograph

El·gi·loy

El·li·ott
    E. femoral condyle blade
        plate

El·lip·ti·cut in·stru·men·ta·
tion

El·lis
    E. procedure

El·lis Jones
    E.J. procedure

El·li·son
    E. procedure

Elms·lie
    E.-Cholmeley procedure

Elms·lie *(continued)*
  E.-Trillat method
  E.-Trillat procedure

elon·ga·tion

ELPS
  excessive lateral pressure
    syndrome

Ely
  E's sign
  E's test

ema·ci·a·tion

em·bole

em·bo·lia

em·bo·lism
  fat e.
  intraosseous fat e.

em·bo·lus *pl.* em·bo·li

EMG
  electromyography

em·i·nence
  antithenar e.
  bicipital e.
  capitate e.
  coccygeal e.
  cochlear e. of sacral bone
  cuneiform e. of head of rib
  deltoid e.
  gluteal e. of femur
  e. of humerus
  hypothenar e.
  iliopectineal e.
  iliopubic e.
  intercondylar e.
  intercondyloid e.
  intermediate e.
  oblique e. of cuboid bone
  radial e. of wrist
  thenar e.
  trochlear e.
  ulnar e. of wrist

em·i·nen·tia *pl.* em·i·nen·
tiae
  e. capitata
  e. carpi radialis
  e. carpi ulnaris
  e. frontale
  e. hypothenaris
  e. iliopectinea
  e. iliopubica
  e. intercondylaris
  e. thenaris

em·py·e·ma
  e. articuli

en·ar·thri·tis

en·ar·thro·di·al

en·ar·thro·sis

en·case·ment

en·chon·dral

en·chon·dro·ma
  multiple congenital e.

en·chon·dro·ma·to·sis
  multiple e.
  skeletal e.

en·chon·dro·ma·tous

en·chon·dro·sis

en·croach·ment

end·chon·dral

En·der
  E. nail

en·do·chon·dral

En·do-Mod·el pros·the·sis

en·do·mys·i·um

en·do·skel·e·ton

en·dos·te·al

en·dos·te·itis

en·dos·te·um

en·dos·ti·tis

en·do·ten·din·e·um

en·do·ten·on

end plate, end-plate
    motor e.p.
    vertebral e.p.

en·er·gy
    kinetic e.
    potential e.
    strain e.

Eng·el·mann
    Camurati-E. syndrome
    E's disease
    E's disk

Eng·en
    E. extension orthosis
    E. palmar basic wrist
        splint
    E. reciprocal orthosis

Engh
    E. fixation score
    E. total hip replacement

en·gi·neer
    rehabilitation e.

En·ne·king
    E. procedure

en·os·to·sis

en·sis·ter·num

ent·epi·con·dyle

en·the·sis

en·the·si·tis

en·the·so·path·ic

en·the·sop·a·thy

en·to·chon·dros·to·sis

en·to·cne·mi·al

en·to·cu·ne·i·form

ent·os·to·sis

en·trap·ment
    popliteal e.

enu·cle·ate

enu·cle·at·ed

enu·cle·a·tion

EO
    elbow orthosis

Eos
    eosinophils

epen·dy·mo·ma

epi·cen·tral

epi·con·dy·lal·gia

epi·con·dyle
    external e. of femur
    external e. of humerus
    internal e. of femur
    internal e. of humerus
    lateral e. of femur
    lateral e. of humerus
    medial e. of femur
    medial e. of humerus

epi·con·dyl·i·an

epi·con·dyl·ic

epi·con·dy·li·tis
    external humeral e.
    lateral e.
    medial e.
    radiohumeral e.

epi·con·dy·lus *pl.* epi·con·dy·
li
    e. lateralis femoris
    e. lateralis humeri
    e. medialis femoris
    e. medialis humeri

epi·cor·a·coid

epi·cos·tal

epi·du·rog·ra·phy

epi·mys·i·ot·omy

epi·mys·i·um

epi·neu·ral

epi·phys·e·al

epi·phys·ec·to·my

epi·phys·i·al

epi·phys·i·od·e·sis
    phalangeal e.

epi·phys·i·oid

epi·phys·i·ol·y·sis

epi·phys·i·om·e·ter

epi·phys·i·op·a·thy

epiph·y·sis *pl.* epiph·y·ses
    capital e.
    opened epiphyses
    slipped e.
    slipped capital femoral e.
    stippled epiphyses

epiph·y·si·tis
    e. juvenilis
    vertebral e.

epi·pyr·a·mis

epi·ro·tu·li·an

L'Epi·scope Za·cha·ry
    L'E.Z. procedure

epi·ster·nal

epi·stro·phe·us

epi·taxy

epi·ten·din·e·um

epi·te·non

epi·the·li·um
    false e.

epith·e·sis

epi·tri·que·trum

epi·troch·lea

E.P. My·cin

ep·o·nych·i·um

Ep·stein
    E. classification (for ante-
      rior dislocation of the
      hip)

Ep·stein *(continued)*
    E. classification (for frac-
      tures associated with hip
      dislocation)
    E. reverse-angle curette

equi·lib·ri·um
    postural e.

equi·no·val·gus

equi·no·va·rus

equi·nus
    ankle e.
    forefoot e.
    gastrocnemius e.
    metatarsus e.

equip·ment
    adaptive e.
    assistive e.
    assistive/adaptive e.

Erb
    E's atrophy
    E's disease
    E's dystrophy
    E's palsy
    E's paralysis
    E.-Goldflam disease

er·go·cal·cif·er·ol

Erich·sen
    E. sign

Ericks·son
    E. procedure
    E. unconstrained device

ero·sion
    endosteal e.

er·y·the·ma

Esch·e·rich·ia
    E. coli

Es·co·bar
    E. syndrome

ESIN
    elastic stable intramedul-
      lary nailing

Es·march
    E. bandage

es·quil·lec·to·my

ESR
    erythrocyte sedimentation
        rate

Es·ser
    E. skin graft

Es·sex
    E.-Lopresti fracture
    E.-Lopresti procedure

es·the·sia

Es·ti·nyl

Es·trace

Es·tra-D

es·tra·di·ol

Es·tra-L

Es·tra·nol-LA

Es·tra·tab

Es·tra·val

Es·tro-Cyp

Es·tro·fem

es·tro·gen

Es·tro·ject

Es·trone

Es·tro·nol

es·tro·pi·pate

Eth·i·bond su·ture

eth·i·nyl es·tra·di·ol

eti·dro·nate

eti·ol·o·gy

eto·do·lac

eval·u·a·tion
    muscle e.
    physical capacities e.

eval·u·a·tion *(continued)*
    Smith physical
        capacities e.

Ev·ans
    E. classification (for intra-
        trochanteric femoral
        fractures)
    E. procedure

ever·sion

evert

ever·tor
    dorsal e's

Ev·o·lu·tion Total Hip Sys·tem

Ewald
    E. elbow prosthesis

EWHO
    elbow-wrist-hand orthosis

Ew·ing
    E's sarcoma
    E's tumor

ex·ac·er·ba·tion

Ex·act-Fit ATH sys·tem

ex·am·i·na·tion
    dark-field microscopic e.
    tendon reflex e.
    vibratory sense e.
    x-ray e.

ex·ar·tic·u·la·tion

Ex·ced·rin

ex·cise

ex·ci·sion
    digital e.
    disk e.
    double metacarpal e.
    nubbin e.

ex·cres·cence

Ex·dol

ex·er·cise
    active-assistive range of
      motion e.
    active range of motion e.
    aerobic e.
    anaerobic e.
    Codman's e.
    Codman pendulum e's
    DeLorme's e.
    eccentric lengthening e.
    extension e's
    flexion e's
    isokinetic e.
    isometric e.
    isotonic e.
    McKenzie e.
    McKenzie extension e.
    passive range of motion e.
    passive resistance e.
    physical therapy e.
    pulley e.
    range of motion e.
    ROM e.
    stretching e's
    weight-bearing e.
    Williams flexion e's

Ex·e·ter
    E. total hip replacement

exo·mys·i·um

ex·os·tec·to·my

ex·os·to·sec·to·my

ex·os·to·sis *pl.* ex·os·to·ses
    e. bursata
    cuneiform e.
    epiphyseal e.
    hereditary multiple exos-
      toses
    hypertrophic e.
    ivory e.
    metatarsal cuneiform e.
    multiple cartilaginous ex-
      ostoses
    multiple exostoses
    retrocalcaneal e.

ex·os·tot·ic

ex·plo·ra·tion

ex·ten·sion
    e. aid
    Boyes finger e.
    Boyes wrist e.
    Buck's e.
    compressive e.
    distractive e.
    dorsal e.
    finger e.
    halo e.
    radial e.
    thoracic e.
    ulnar e.

ex·ten·sor
    e. carpi radialis brevis
    e. carpi radialis longus
    e. carpi ulnaris
    e. digiti quinti proprius
    e. digitorum brevis
    e. digitorum communis
    e. digitorum longus
    extrinsic finger e's
    extrinsic wrist e.
    finger e's
    e. hallucis brevis
    e. hallucis longus
    e. indicis proprius
    e. pollicis brevis
    e. pollicis longus
    toe e.

ex·tir·pa·tion

ex·tra-ar·tic·u·lar

ex·tra·car·pal

ex·tract

ex·trac·tion

ex·trac·tor
    driver-bender-e.
    driver-e.
    femoral head e.
    e.-impactor
    impactor-e.
    Küntscher e.
    Massie e.

ex·trac·tor *(continued)*
    Moore prosthesis e.
    staple e.

ex·trac·tor-im·pac·tor
    Fox e.-i.

ex·tra·epi·phys·e·al

ex·tra·fo·ram·i·nal

ex·tra·lig·a·men·tous

ex·tra·mal·le·o·lus

ex·tra·mas·toi·di·tis

ex·tra·med·ul·la·ry

ex·tra·os·se·ous

ex·tra·pel·vic

ex·tra·peri·os·te·al

ex·tra·plan·tar

ex·tra·skel·e·tal

ex·tra·spi·nal

ex·tra·sy·no·vi·al

ex·trem·i·tas *pl.* ex·trem·i·ta·tes
    e. acromialis claviculae
    e. sternalis claviculae

ex·trem·i·ty
    cartilaginous e. of rib
    external e. of clavicle
    internal e. of clavicle
    proximal e. of phalanx of
      finger
    proximal e. of phalanx of
      toe
    scapular e. of clavicle

ex·u·date

Ey·ler
    E. procedure

Fa·ber
F. maneuver
F. test

fac·et
articular f.
articular f. of atlas, circular
articular f. of atlas, inferior
articular f. of atlas, superior
articular f. of axis, anterior
articular f's for rib cartilages
f. of calcaneus, posterior, medial
clavicular f.
costal f., anterior
costal f., inferior
costal f., posterior
costal f., superior
costal f's of sternum
costal f. of vertebra, superior
fibular f.
lateral f. of patella
lateral f's of sternum
locked f.
locked f's of spine
malleolar f. of tibia, internal
f's of patella
proximal tibiofibular f.
f. of spine
squatting f.
f. for tubercle of rib

fac·e·tec·to·my

fa·ci·es *pl.* fa·ci·es
f. anterior lateralis humeri
f. anterior medialis humeri

fa·ci·es *(continued)*
f. anterior patellae
f. anterior radii
f. anterior scapulae
f. anterior ulnae
f. anterolateralis humeri
f. anteromedialis humeri
f. articularis acromialis claviculae
f. articularis acromialis scapulae
f. articularis acromii scapulae
f. articularis anterior axis
f. articularis anterior calcanei
f. articularis anterior epistrophei
f. articularis calcanea anterior tali
f. articularis calcanea media tali
f. articularis calcanea posterior tali
f. articularis capitis costae
f. articularis capitis fibulae
f. articularis capituli costae
f. articularis capituli fibulae
f. articularis carpalis radii
f. articularis carpea radii
f. articularis carpi radii
f. articularis cuboidea calcanei
f. articularis fibularis tibiae
f. articulares inferiores atlantis
f. articularis inferior tibiae
f. articulares inferiores vertebrarum

fa·ci·es *(continued)*
- f. articularis malleolaris tibiae
- f. articularis malleoli fibulae
- f. articularis media calcanei
- f. articularis navicularis tali
- f. articularis patellae
- f. articularis posterior axis
- f. articularis sternalis claviculae
- f. articularis superior tibiae
- f. articularis talaris anterior calcanei
- f. articularis talaris media calcanei
- f. articularis talaris posterior calcanei
- f. articularis tuberculi costae
- f. auricularis ossis ilium
- f. auricularis ossis sacri
- f. costalis scapulae
- f. digitales
- f. digitales dorsales manus
- f. digitales dorsales pedis
- f. digitales fibulares pedis
- f. digitales laterales manus
- f. digitales laterales pedis
- f. digitales mediales manus
- f. digitales mediales pedis
- f. digitales palmares manus
- f. digitales plantares pedis
- f. digitales radiales manus
- f. digitales tibiales pedis
- f. digitales ulnares manus
- f. digitales ventrales manus
- f. digitales ventrales pedis
- f. dorsalis ossis sacri
- f. dorsalis radii
- f. dorsalis scapulae

fa·ci·es *(continued)*
- f. dorsalis ulnae
- f. glutea ossis ilii
- f. lateralis fibulae
- f. lateralis radii
- f. lateralis tibiae
- f. lunata acetabuli
- f. malleolaris lateralis tali
- f. malleolaris medialis tali
- f. medialis fibulae
- f. medialis tibiae
- f. medialis ulnae
- f. patellaris femoris
- f. pelvica ossis sacri
- f. pelvina ossis sacri
- f. poplitea femoris
- f. posterior fibulae
- f. posterior humeri
- f. posterior radii
- f. posterior scapulae
- f. posterior tibiae
- f. posterior ulnae
- f. sacropelvina ossis ilii
- f. superior trochleae tali
- f. symphyseos ossis pubis
- f. symphysialis
- f. ventralis scapulae
- f. volaris radii
- f. volaris ulnae

F-act·in

fac·tor
- antinuclear f. (ANF)
- heparin-binding fibroblast growth f.
- instability f.
- insulin-like growth f's (IGF)
- platelet-derived growth f.
- RA f.
- rheumatoid f. (RF)
- skeletal growth f.

Fa·hey
- F. and O'Brien procedure

fail·ure
- brittle f.
- ductile f.

fail·ure *(continued)*
    fatigue f.
    f. of segmentation of verte-
        bra

Fair·banks
    F. changes
    F. and Sever procedure

Fa·jer·sztajn
    F. crossed sciatic sign

falx *pl.* fal·ces
    aponeurotic f.
    f. aponeurotica
    inguinal f.
    f. inguinalis
    f. ligamentosa
    ligamentous f.

Fan·co·ni
    F's anemia
    F's pancytopenia syndrome
    F. syndrome

Far·a·beuf
    F's amputation

Far·ber
    Warner and F. procedure

Farm·er
    F. procedure

Far·rar
    McKee-F. total hip re-
        placement

fas·cia *pl.* fas·ciae
    Abernethy's f.
    antebrachial f.
    f. antebrachii
    f. of arm
    f. axillaris
    bicipital f.
    brachial f.
    f. brachialis
    f. brachii
    cervical f.
    cervical f., deep
    f. cervicalis
    clavipectoral f.

fas·cia *(continued)*
    f. clavipectoralis
    Cloquet's f.
    f. colli
    coracoclavicular f.
    f. coracoclavicularis
    coracocostal f.
    cribriform f.
    f. cribrosa
    crural f.
    f. cruris
    deep f. of arm
    deep f. of back
    deep f. of forearm
    deep f. of thigh
    deltoid f.
    f. deltoidea
    dorsal f., deep
    dorsal f. of foot
    dorsal f. of hand
    f. dorsalis manus
    f. dorsalis pedis
    femoral f.
    f. of forearm
    iliac f.
    f. iliaca
    f. iliopectinea
    iliopectineal f.
    f. lata femoris
    f. of leg
    longitudinal f., anterior
    longitudinal f., posterior
    lumbodorsal f.
    f. lumbodorsalis
    f. of nape
    f. of neck
    f. nuchae
    nuchal f.
    f. nuchalis
    obturator f.
    f. obturatoria
    palmar f.
    parietal f. of pelvis
    f. pectinea
    pectineal f.
    pectoral f.
    f. pectoralis
    pelvic f., parietal

fas·cia *(continued)*
    f. pelvica parietalis
    f. pelvis parietalis
    plantar f.
    prevertebral f.
    f. prevertebralis
    proper f. of neck
    f. propria colli
    scalene f.
    semilunar f.
    Sibson's f.
    f. of thigh
    f. thoracolumbalis
    triangular f. of abdomen
    triangular f. of Quain
    volar f.

fas·cial

fas·cia·plas·ty

fas·ci·cle

fas·cic·u·lus *pl.* fas·cic·cu·li
    f. exilis
    fibrous f. of biceps muscle
    longitudinal fasciculi of
        cruciform ligament
    fasciculi longitudinales li-
        gamenti cruciformis at-
        lantis
    fasciculi transversi apo-
        neurosis palmaris
    fasciculi transversi apo-
        neurosis plantaris

fas·ci·ec·to·my
    palmar f.

fas·ci·itis
    nodular f.

fas·ci·od·e·sis

fas·cio·gram

fas·cio·plas·ty

fas·ci·or·rha·phy

fas·ci·ot·o·my
    palmar f.

fat
    Hoffa f.

fa·tigue
    muscle f.

FBS
    fasting blood sugar

feb·rile

feet

Feil
    Klippel-F. sequence

Feiss
    F's line

Fel·dene

fel·on
    aseptic f.

Fel·ty
    F's syndrome

Fem·i·none

Fem·o·gen

Fem·o·gex

fem·o·ra

fem·o·ral

fem·o·ro·il·i·ac

fem·o·ro·tib·i·al

fe·mur *pl.* fem·o·ra
    head of f.
    neck of f.
    subtrochanteric f.

fen·es·trate

fen·o·pro·fen

Fer·gu·son
    F. reduction
    F. view
    F.-Thompson osteotomy

Fer·gus·son
    F. method for measuring
        scoliosis

Fer·ré
  Sorrondo-F. amputation

Fer·ris
  F.-Smith rongeur

FES
  functional electrical stim-
    ulation

FFP
  fresh frozen plasma

FG syn·drome

FI
  fibula, complete (congeni-
    tal absence of limb)

fi
  fibula, incomplete (congen-
    ital absence of limb)

fi·ber
  asbestos f's
  bone f's
  carbon f.
  dark f's
  extrafusal f's
  Gerdy's f's
  intrafusal f's
  Kaplan's f's
  light f's
  muscle f.
  muscle f's, fast twitch
  muscle f's, slow twitch
  muscle f's, type I
  muscle f's, type II
  osteocollagenous f's
  osteogenetic f's
  osteogenic f's
  radiating f's of anterior
    chondrosternal ligaments
  Sharpey's f's
  Weissmann's f's

fi·bra pl. fi·brae
  fibrae annulares
  muscular f.

fi·bril
  muscle f.

fi·bril·la·tion

fi·bro·blast

fi·bro·car·ti·lage
  circumferential f.
  connecting f.
  cotyloid f.
  elastic f.
  interarticular f.
  intervertebral f's
  semilunar f's
  spongy f.
  stratiform f.
  white f.
  yellow f.

fi·bro·car·ti·lag·i·nous

fi·bro·car·ti·la·go pl. fi·bro·
  car·ti·lag·i·nes
  fibrocartilagines interver-
    tebrales
  f. navicularis

fi·bro·chon·dri·tis

fi·bro·chon·dro·gen·e·sis

fi·bro·cyte

fi·bro·dys·pla·sia

fi·bro·fas·ci·tis

fi·bro·gen·e·sis
  f. imperfecta ossium

fi·bro·ma
  f. of bone
  chondromyxoid f.
  desmoplastic f.
  desmoplastic f. of bone
  nonossifying f.
  nonossifying f. of bone
  nonosteogenic f.
  ossifying f. of long bone
  periosteal f.

fi·bro·ma·to·sis
  congenital f.
  palmar f.
  plantar f.

fi·bro·my·itis

fi·bro·myo·si·tis
  nodular f.

fi·bro·plate

fi·bro·sar·co·ma

fi·bro·sis

fi·bro·si·tis
  periarticular f.

fi·bro·xan·tho·ma

fi·bro·xan·tho·sar·co·ma

fib·u·la
  collateral sprain of f.
  neck of f.

fib·u·lar

fib·u·la·ris

fib·u·lec·to·my

fib·u·lo·cal·ca·ne·al

Fi·cat
  F. classification (for avas-
    cular necrosis)
  F's projection

fi·dic·i·na·les

field
  Cohnheim's f's
  magnetic f.

Field·ing
  F. classification (for sub-
    trochanteric fractures of
    the femur)

fil·a·ment
  desmin f's

Fi·li·piu
  Baciu and F. arthrodesis

fill·er

film
  baseline f.
  flexion-extension f.
  scout f.

film *(continued)*
  toe f.

fi·lum *pl.* fi·la
  f. terminale

fin·ger
  arthrodesis f.
  baseball f.
  drop f.
  first f.
  football f.
  giant f.
  hammer f.
  hippocratic f's
  index f.
  lock f.
  mallet f.
  movement of f.
  ring f.
  snapping f.
  spring f.
  sublimis f.
  trigger f.

Fin·kel·stein
  F. sign
  F's test

Fisch·er
  Ace-F. fixation device
  F. rasp

Fish·er
  Abbott-F.-Lucas arthro-
    desis
  F. guide

Fiske & Sub·ba·Row re·duc·
er

fis·tu·la *pl.* fis·tu·lae, fis·tu·
las
  arteriovenous f.

fit·ting
  immediate postsurgical f.

fix·ate

fix·a·teur

fix·a·tion
    AO internal f.
    bicortical f.
    biodegradable f.
    bolt f.
    cancellous f.
    cerclage f.
    cortical f.
    dorsal plate f.
    external f.
    external skeleton f.
    fracture f.
    graft f.
    hook-pin f.
    internal f.
    intraosseous f.
    K-wire f.
    open reduction and inter-
        nal f. (ORIF)
    pedicle f.
    pedicle screw f.
    plate f.
    postural f.
    rotary f.
    screw f.
    segmental f.
    skeletal f.
    sleeve-sublaminar f.
    Zickel f.

fix·a·tor
    Ace-Fischer f.
    Calandruccio external f.
    external f.
    Rezaian spinal f.

flac·cid

Flag·yl

flail

flair
    lateral trochanteric f.

Fla·na·gan
    F. and Burem graft

flap
    Atosoy f.
    cross-finger f.

flap *(continued)*
    delayed f.
    extensor retinaculum f.
    fasciocutaneous f.
    fingertip f.
    island pedicle f.
    Kutler f.
    pedicle f.
    rotational f.
    thenar f.
    tumbler f.
    Wolfe-graft f.

flat·foot
    congenital rocker-bottom f.
    peroneal spastic f.
    rocker-bottom f.
    spastic f.

Flatt
    F. driver
    F. finger/thumb prosthesis
    F. prosthesis
    F. self-retaining screw-
        driver

fla·vec·to·my

flec·tion

Fleisch·ner
    F's disease

flex

flex·i·bil·i·ty

flex·ion
    active f.
    Boyes finger f.
    Brand finger f.
    Bunnell finger f.
    compressive f.
    distractive f.
    finger f.
    Fowler finger f.
    hip f.
    lateral f.
    palmar f.
    plantar f.
    Pulver-Taft finger f.

flex·ion *(continued)*
    Riordan finger f.
    Stiles-Bunnell finger f.

flex·ion-com·pres·sion

flex·ion-dis·trac·tion

flex·or
    f. carpi radialis
    f. carpi ulnaris
    f. digiti quinti
    f. digitorum brevis
    f. digitorum longus
    f. digitorum profundus
    f. digitorum sublimis
    f. digitorum superficialis
    extrinsic finger f's
    extrinsic wrist f.
    finger f.
    f. hallucis brevis
    f. pollicis longus
    f. retinaculum
    wrist f.

flex·or·plas·ty
    Steindler f.

flex·ure
    lumbar f.

Floe·gel
    F's layer

Flood
    F's ligament

flo·ra
    common f.

Flor·i·da brace

flow
    transsynovial f.

flu·id
    synovial f.

flu·o·ros·co·py

flu·o·ro·sis

Flu·o·ro-Zyme

flur·bip·ro·fen

FNA
    fine-needle aspiration

FNS
    functional neuromuscular
        stimulation

FO
    foot orthosis

Fo
    forearm amputation

fo·cil, fo·cile

Foix
    Marie-F. sign

fold
    alar f's
    interarticular f. of hip
    medial synovial f.
    nail f.
    synovial f.
    synovial f., infrapatellar
    synovial f., patellar
    synovial f. of hip

Fo·lex

Fo·lex PFS

foot
    athlete's f.
    broad f.
    cavus f.
    Charcot's f.
    cleft f.
    club f.
    Egyptian f.
    energy-storing f.
    flat f.
    forced f.
    Friedreich's f.
    Greek f.
    hypermobile flat f. with
        tight tendo Achillis
        (HFFTTA)
    march f.
    Morton's f.
    multiaxial f.
    f. orthosis

foot *(continued)*
  prosthetic f.
  rear f.
  reel f.
  rocker-bottom f.
  SACH (solid ankle cushion heel) f.
  SAFE (stationary attachment flexible endoskeletal) f.
  sag f.
  single-axis f.
  spread f.
  subtalar f.
  tabetic f.
  taut f.
  weak f.

foot·print

fo·ra·men *pl.* fo·ra·mi·na
  arterial f.
  f. costotransversarium
  costotransverse f.
  cotyloid f.
  Hartigan's f.
  infrapiriform f.
  intersacral foramina
  intervertebral f.
  f. intervertebrale
  foramina intervertebralia ossis sacri
  intervertebral foramina of sacrum
  ischiadic f., greater
  ischiadic f., lesser
  f. ischiadicum majus
  f. ischiadicum minus
  ischiopubic f.
  f. magnum
  medullary f.
  neural f.
  f. nutricium
  f. nutriens
  nutrient f.
  obturator f.
  f. obturatorium
  f. obturatum
  oval f. of hip bone

fo·ra·men *(continued)*
  f. processus transversi
  sacral foramina, anterior
  sacral foramina, dorsal
  sacral foramina, internal
  sacral foramina, posterior
  sacral foramina, ventral
  f. of sacral canal
  foramina sacralia anteriora
  foramina sacralia dorsalia
  foramina sacralia pelvica
  foramina sacralia pelvina
  foramina sacralia posteriora
  foramina sacralia ventralia
  sacrosciatic f., great
  sacrosciatic f., small
  f. of saphenous vein
  sciatic f., greater
  sciatic f., lesser
  f. sciaticum majus
  f. sciaticum minus
  spinal f.
  f. of spinal cord
  suprapiriform f.
  thyroid f.
  f. transversarium
  foramina venarum minimarum atrii dextri
  vertebral f.
  f. vertebrale
  vertebroarterial f.
  f. vertebroarteriale
  Weitbrecht's f.

fo·ram·i·na

fo·ram·i·not·o·my
  partial f.

Forbes
  F. procedure

force
  offset loading f.
  rotational f.
  tilting f.

for·ceps
>   Backhaus towel f.
>   bone cutting f.
>   bone holding f.
>   Kern bone holding f.
>   Lane bone holding f.
>   ligamenta flava f.
>   micropituitary f.
>   plain tissue f.
>   rongeur f.
>   sequestrum f.
>   Stille-Liston bone
>   cutting f.
>   straight flexible f.
>   tissue f.
>   toothed tissue f.
>   towel f.
>   upbiting f.

fore·arm

fore·fin·ger

fore·foot
>   pronated f.
>   valgus f.

fore·quar·ter

Fo·res·tier
>   F. disease

for·ma·tion
>   marginal osteophyte f.

for·mu·la *pl.* for·mu·lae, for·
mu·las
>   digital f.
>   vertebral f.

Forss·man
>   Börjeson-F.-Lehmann syn-
>   drome

For·taz

fos·sa *pl.* fos·sae
>   acetabular f.
>   f. acetabuli
>   anconal f.
>   anconeal f.
>   antecubital f.

fos·sa *(continued)*
>   articular f. of atlas, infe-
>   rior
>   articular f. of atlas, supe-
>   rior
>   articular f. for odontoid
>   process of axis
>   articular f. of temporal
>   bone
>   f. capitis femoris
>   condyloid f. of atlas
>   f. coronoidea humeri
>   coronoid f. of humerus
>   f. of coronoid process
>   costal f., inferior
>   costal f., superior
>   costal f. of transverse proc-
>   ess
>   cubital f.
>   f. cubitalis
>   digital f. of femur
>   glenoid f.
>   glenoid f. of scapula
>   Gruber's f.
>   f. of head of femur
>   iliac f.
>   f. iliaca
>   f. infraspinata
>   intercondylar f. of femur
>   intercondylar f. of femur,
>   anterior
>   intercondylar f. of tibia,
>   anterior
>   intercondylar f. of tibia,
>   posterior
>   f. intercondylaris femoris
>   f. intercondylica
>   intercondyloid f.
>   f. intercondyloidea ante-
>   rior tibiae
>   f. intercondyloidea femoris
>   f. intercondyloidea poste-
>   rior tibiae
>   Jobert's f.
>   f. of lateral malleolus
>   f. of little head of radius
>   f. malleoli lateralis
>   f. olecrani

fos·sa *(continued)*
    olecranon f.
    f. ovalis femoris
    oval f. of thigh
    patellar f. of femur
    patellar f. of tibia
    f. poplitea
    popliteal f. of femur
    popliteal f. of tibia
    posterior f. of humerus
    prescapular f.
    prespinous f.
    radial f. of humerus
    f. radialis humeri
    rhomboid f.
    semilunar f. of ulna
    sigmoid f. of ulna
    sigmoid f. of ulna, lesser
    subscapular f.
    f. subscapularis
    supracondyloid f.
    f. supraspinata
    supraspinous f.
    supratrochlear f., posterior
    tibiofemoral f.
    trochanteric f.
    f. trochanterica
    ulnar f.

fos·su·la *pl.* fos·su·lae
    costal f., inferior
    costal f., superior

Fos·ter
    F. frame
    Siffert-F.-Nachamie procedure

Four·ni·er
    F. test

fo·vea *pl.* fo·veae
    anterior f. of humerus, greater
    anterior f. of humerus, lesser
    articular foveae for rib cartilages
    f. articularis capitis radii

fo·vea *(continued)*
    f. articularis inferior atlantis
    f. articularis superior atlantis
    calcaneal f.
    f. capitis femoris
    f. capituli radii
    f. of coronoid process
    costal f., inferior
    costal f., superior
    costal f., transverse
    costal foveae of sternum
    f. costalis inferior
    f. costalis processus transversus
    f. costalis superior
    dental f. of atlas
    f. dentis atlantis
    f. of head of femur
    f. for head of radius
    inferior articular f. of atlas
    f. of lateral malleolus
    f. of little head of radius
    malleolar f., lateral, of fibula
    supratrochlear f., anterior
    supratrochlear f. of humerus
    f. of talus
    f. of tooth of atlas

Fow·ler
    F. arthroplasty
    F. finger flexion
    F. maneuver
    F. opponensplasty
    F. procedure
    F. release

Fowles
    F. procedure

Fox
    F. extractor-impactor
    F. internal fixation device
    F.-Blazina procedure

Foy·gen Aq·ue·ous

FPB
   femoropopliteal bypass

frac·tog·ra·phy

frac·ture
   abduction f.
   adduction f.
   agenetic f.
   anatomic neck f.
   angulation of f.
   apophyseal f.
   articular f.
   articular pillar f.
   articular process f.
   atrophic f.
   avulsion f.
   backfire f.
   Barton's f.
   basal neck f.
   basocervical f.
   bending f.
   Bennett's f.
   bicondylar f.
   bimalleolar f.
   bipedicular f.
   boot-top f.
   Bosworth f.
   bowing f.
   boxer's f.
   bucket-handle f.
   bumper f.
   burst f.
   bursting f.
   butterfly f.
   buttonhole f.
   cartwheel f.
   central f.
   Chance f.
   chauffeur's f.
   chip f.
   chisel f.
   clay-shoveler's f.
   cleavage f.
   closed f.
   Colles' f.
   combination f.
   comminuted f.
   complete f.

frac·ture *(continued)*
   complicated f.
   compound f.
   compression f.
   condylar f.
   cortical f.
   cotton f.
   crush f.
   D/3 f.
   Darrach-Hugston-Milch f.
   dashboard f.
   dens f.
   dentate f.
   depressed f.
   de Quervain's f.
   diacondylar f.
   direct f.
   dislocation f.
   displaced f.
   distal f.
   distal/3 f.
   dome f.
   double f.
   Dupuytren's f.
   Duverney's f.
   dyscrasic f.
   f. en coin
   endocrine f.
   f. en rave
   epicondylar f.
   epiphyseal f.
   epiphyseal slip f.
   Essex-Lopresti f.
   extracapsular f.
   facet f.
   fatigue f.
   fender f.
   fissure f.
   fissured f.
   four-part f.
   Galeazzi's f.
   Gosselin's f.
   greenstick f.
   grenade-thrower's f.
   hairline f.
   hangman's f.
   Hermodsson f.
   hickory-stick f.

frac·ture *(continued)*
- high dens f.
- Hill-Sachs f.
- Hohl f.
- idiopathic f.
- impacted f.
- impaction f.
- incomplete f.
- indirect f.
- inflammatory f.
- infraction f.
- insufficiency f.
- interperiosteal f.
- intertrochanteric f.
- intra-articular f.
- intracapsular f.
- intraperiosteal f.
- inversion stress f.
- Jefferson f.
- joint f.
- Jones f.
- Kocher f.
- laminar f.
- lead pipe f.
- Le Fort's f.
- linear f.
- Lisfranc's f.
- longitudinal f.
- loose f.
- lorry driver's f.
- low dens f.
- M/3 f.
- Maisonneuve f.
- Malgaigne f.
- mallet f.
- malunited f.
- march f.
- middle f.
- middle/3 f.
- Monteggia's f.
- Montercaux f.
- Moore's f.
- multiple f.
- multizonal f.
- f. of necessity
- neoplastic f.
- neurogenic f.
- nightstick f.

frac·ture *(continued)*
- nondisplaced f.
- oblique f.
- occult f.
- odontoid f.
- olecranon f.
- one-part f.
- open f.
- osteoporotic f.
- P/3 f.
- paratrooper f.
- parry f.
- patellar f.
- pathologic f.
- perforating f.
- periarticular f.
- periprosthetic f.
- pertrochanteric f.
- Piedmont f.
- pillion f.
- plafond f.
- plastic bowing f.
- posterior element f.
- Pott's f.
- pressure f.
- proximal f.
- Quervain's f.
- resecting f.
- reverse Barton f.
- reverse Colles' f.
- ring f.
- Roland f.
- Rolando f.
- Salter f. (I–VI)
- Salter-Harris f.
- scaphoid f.
- secondary f.
- segmental f.
- Segond f.
- shaft f.
- Shepherd's f.
- short bone f.
- shoulder f.
- silver-fork f.
- simple f.
- simple f., complex
- Skillern's f.
- Smith's f.

frac·ture *(continued)*
  spinal f. (Types I–III)
  spine f.
  spiral f.
  splintered f.
  spontaneous f.
  sprain f.
  Springer's f.
  sprinter's f.
  stellate f.
  Stieda's f.
  straddle f.
  stress f.
  subcapital f.
  subchondral f.
  subcutaneous f.
  subperiosteal f.
  subtrochanteric f.
  supracondylar f.
  surgical neck f.
  T f.
  f. table
  teardrop f.
  three-part f.
  tibial plateau f.
  tibial spine f.
  Tillaux Kleiger f.
  torsion f.
  torus f.
  transcervical f.
  transcondylar f.
  transverse f.
  trimalleolar f.
  triplane f.
  trochanteric f.
  tuft f.
  two-part f.
  undisplaced f.
  unstable f.
  ununited f.
  vertebra plana f.
  Volkmann f.
  wagon wheel f.
  Wagstaffe's f.
  Weber f.
  wedge f.
  wedge compression f.
  willow f.

frac·ture *(continued)*
  Y f.

frac·ture-dis·lo·ca·tion
  f.d. of ankle
  Monteggia f.d.

frac·ture-sep·a·ra·tion

fra·gil·i·tas
  f. ossium
  f. ossium congenita

fra·gil·i·ty
  hereditary f. of bone

frag·ment
  displaced f.
  distal f.
  fracture f.
  free disk f.
  proximal f.
  retained f.
  sequestrated disk f.
  undisplaced f.

frame
  Balkan f.
  Böhler-Braun f.
  Bradford f.
  claw-type basic f.
  Foster f.
  Heffington f.
  IV-type basic f.
  Jones abduction f.
  radiolucent f.
  spinal surgery f.
  Stryker f.
  Whitman's f.
  Wingfield f.

Frän·kel
  F. classification
  F. line
  F. neurological assessment
  F. sign

Frank Dick·son
  F.D. shelf procedure

Fra·ser
  F. syndrome

Free·man
F. resurfacing procedure
F. total hip replacement
F.-Sheldon syndrome
F.-Swanson unconstrained device

Freer
F. elevator
F. elevator-dissector

Frei·berg
F's disease
F's infraction

Frej·ka
F. orthosis
F. pillow splint

French
F. osteotomy
F. procedure

fre·num *pl.* fre·na
Macdowel's f.

fresh·en·ing

fri·a·ble

fric·tion
coefficient of f.

Fried
F. and Green procedure

Frie·dreich
F's ataxia
F's foot

Fro·ben

Fröh·lich
Babinski-F. syndrome
F. adiposogenital dystrophy

Froim·son
F. and Oh procedure

Fro·ment
F. paper sign
f. cranii

front
corset f.

Fro·riep
F's induration

Frosst·image MDP

Frosst·image Sul·fur Col·loid

Frost
F. procedure
Majestro, Ruda, and F. procedure

frost·bite

Fryk·man
fracture classification system

FTSG
full-thickness skin graft

Fu·ci·din

ful·gu·ra·tion

Ful·ker·son
F. procedure

fu·nic·u·lus *pl.* fu·nic·u·li
ligamentous f.

fu·nis
f. hippocratis

fu·si·dic acid

fu·si·form

fu·sion
Albee lumbar spinal f.
anterior cervical f.
anterior interbody f.
anterior lumbar body f.
anterior spinal f.
atlantoaxial f.
bilateral lateral f.
bony f.
Bosworth lumbar spinal f.
Compare and Thompson f.
diaphyseal-epiphyseal f.
DIP f.
extraarticular f.

fu·sion *(continued)*
    Gill lumbar spinal f.
    Gill, Manning, and White
      lumbar spinal f.
    Harrington rod f.
    Hibbs spinal f.
    hip f.
    interbody f.
    intraarticular f.
    kneeling lumbar spine f.
    lateral f.
    lumbar intertransverse
      process spinal f.
    occipitocervical f.
    Overton lumbar spinal f.
    pantalar f.
    percutaneous interbody f.
    PIP f.
    posterior f.

fu·sion *(continued)*
    posterior cervical spinal f.
    posterior interbody f.
    posterior lumbar spinal f.
    posterior spinal f.
    posterolateral f.
    posterolateral interbody f.
    postinterlaminar f.
    f. of joint
    Robinson and Riley
      spinal f.
    Robinson and Southwick
      cervical spinal f.
    Roger's f.
    Roger cervical spinal f.
    spinal f.
    subaxial f.
    symmetric f. of vertebra
    Whitecloud and Larocca
      spinal f.

G-ac·tin

Gaens·len
G. sign
G's test

GAG
glycosaminoglycan

gait
antalgic g.
drop-foot g.
dystrophic g.
gluteus maximus g.
gluteus medius g.
slap foot g.
training g.
waddling g.

Ga·lan·te
Harris-G. total hip re-
placement
Harris-G. Porous-Coated
Hip System
Miller-G. (MG) Knee Sys-
tem

Ga·le·az·zi
G.-equivalent lesion
G's fracture
G. lesion
G. sign

Gal·lis
G. procedure

Gal·ves·ton
Luque-G. instrumentation

gam·ma·car·boxy·glu·tam·ic
ac·id

gam·ma glu·ta·myl trans·fer·
ase (GGT)

gam·ma glu·ta·myl trans·
pep·ti·dase

gamma GT

gamp·so·dac·ty·ly

gan·gli·ec·to·my

gan·gli·on *pl.* gan·glia, gan·
gli·ons
Acrel's g.
compound g.
diffuse g.
periosteal g.
primary g.
simple g.
synovial g.
wrist g.

gan·gli·on·ec·to·my

gan·glio·neu·ro·ma

gan·gli·on·ic

gan·gli·on·os·to·my

gan·grene

Gant
G. hip arthrodesis
G. osteotomy

Gan·ta·nol

Ga·ra·my·cin

Gar·ceau
G. procedure

Gar·den
G. fracture classification
system

Gard·ner
G's syndrome
G.-Wells calipers
G.-Wells tongs

Gar·ré
chronic sclerosing osteo-
myelitis of G.
G's disease
G's osteitis
G's osteomyelitis

Gart·land
    Berman and G. procedure

^{67}Ga (gallium) scan

gas·troc·ne·mi·us

Gau·cher
    G's disease
    G's lesions

gauge
    acetabular g.
    bone screw g.
    gap g.
    screw depth g.

gaunt·let
    padded g.

Ge·gen·baur
    G's cell

gel
    agarose g.

Gel·foam

Gel·man
    G. procedure

Gen·e·sis To·tal Knee Sys·tem

ge·nic·u·lar

Gen·pril

gen·ta·mi·cin
    g. sulfate

ge·nu *pl.* ge·nua
    g. extrorsum
    g. impressum
    g. introrsum
    g. recurvatum
    g. valgum
    g. varum

Geo·med·ic un·con·strained de·vice

Ge·rard
    G. resurfacing procedure

Ger·dy
    G's fibers
    G's ligament
    G's tubercle

Ger·old
    Baller-G. syndrome

Get·ty
    G. spine procedure

GGT
    γ-glutamyltransferase

GGTP
    gamma-glutamyltransferase

Ghorm·ley
    G. arthrodesis
    G. osteotomy

Gian·nes·tras
    G. procedure

gib·bos·i·ty

gib·bous

gib·bus
    fracture g.

Gib·ney
    G. bandage
    G's disease
    G's perispondylitis
    G's strapping

Gib·son
    G. technique

Gied·i·on
    Langer-G. syndrome
    Schinzel-G. syndrome

Gi·gli
    G. saw

Gi·li·ber·ty
    G. total hip replacement

Gill
    Abbott and G. osteotomy
    G. arthrodesis
    G. lumbar spinal fusion

Gill *(continued)*
  G. procedure
  G. shelf procedure
  G., Manning, and White
    lumbar spinal fusion
  G.-Stein arthrodesis

Gil·lies
  G. graft
  G. pollicization
  G. and Millard technique

Gim·ber·nat
  reflex ligament of G.

gin·gly·form

gin·gly·mo·ar·thro·di·al

gin·gly·moid

gin·gly·mus

gir·dle
  g. of inferior member
  pectoral g.
  pelvic g.
  shoulder g.
  thoracic g.

Gir·dle·stone
  G. operation
  G. resection
  G.-Taylor procedure

GLA
  gamma-carboxyglutamic
    acid

gla·di·o·lus

gla·dio·ma·nu·bri·al

gland
  haversian g's
  mucilaginous g's
  synovial g's
  thyroid g.

Gla·zer
  Ecker, Lotke, and G. ten-
    don transfer

gle·no·hu·mer·al

gle·noid

gli·o·ma

Glis·son
  G's sling

glob
  globulin

glob·ule
  Dobie's g.

glob·u·lin
  immune serum g.
  g. X

glu·co·sa·mine

glu·teth·i·mide

glu·te·us max·i·mus

glu·te·us me·di·us

glu·te·us min·i·mus

glu·ti·tis

gly·cos·ami·no·gly·can

G-My·cin

gold
  g. sodium thiomalate

Gold·flam
  Erb-G. disease

Gold·mar
  G. opponensplasty

Gold·thwait
  G. sign
  Roux-G. procedure

Gol·gi
  G's corpuscles

Goltz
  G. syndrome

Gom·ori
  G. stain

gon·ag·ra

go·nal·gia

gon·ar·thri·tis

gon·ar·throc·a·ce

gon·ar·thro·men·in·gi·tis

gon·ar·thro·sis

gon·ar·throt·o·my

go·nato·cele

gon·e·itis

go·ni·om·e·ter
 polarized light g.

go·ni·tis
 fungous g.
 g. tuberculosa

gono·camp·sis

gony·camp·sis

gony·cro·te·sis

gony·ec·ty·po·sis

gonyo·cele

gony·on·cus

Gor·don
 G.-Taylor amputation

Gore
 G. AO screw

Gore-Tex

Gor·ham
 G's disease

Gor·lin
 G. syndrome

Gos·se·lin
 G's fracture

Gouf·fon
 G. pin

gouge
 Cobb g.
 curved g.
 gooseneck g.
 Hibbs g.
 Kelley g.
 Meyerding g.

gouge *(continued)*
 Semi-Circular g.
 semicircular g.
 Smith-Petersen g.
 straight g.
 swan neck g.

gout
 abarticular g.
 articular g.
 chalky g.
 idiopathic g.
 irregular g.
 latent g.
 masked g.
 misplaced g.
 oxalic g.
 polyarticular g.
 primary g.
 regular g.
 rheumatic g.
 secondary g.
 tophaceous g.

gou·ty

Gow·er

Gow·ers
 G. sign
 G. type muscular dystro-
 phy

Goy·rand
 G's injury

Gra·ber
 G.-Duvernay procedure

grade
 Risser g.

graft
 Albee g.
 allogenic g.
 allogenous g.
 autochthonous g.
 autogenous g.
 autogenous saphenous
 vein g.
 Banks g.
 Blair-Brown skin g.

graft *(continued)*
- bone g.
- Boyd g.
- Braun skin g.
- Campbell g.
- cancellous g.
- chemosterilized g.
- chip g.
- clothespin g.
- Cloward g.
- composite g.
- cortical g.
- corticocancellous g.
- cross-leg pedicle g.
- Davis skin g.
- demineralized bone g.
- diamond inlay g.
- double skin g.
- Dragstedt skin g.
- dual onlay g.
- Esser skin g.
- extraarticular g.
- fascia lata g.
- fibular g.
- g. fixation
- Flanagan and Burem g.
- free g.
- freeze-dried g.
- full-thickness skin g.
- Gillies g.
- Haldeman g.
- hemicylindric g.
- Henderson g.
- Henry g.
- Hey-Groves-Kirk g.
- Hoaglund g.
- horseshoe g.
- Huntington g.
- ileal strut g.
- iliac g.
- Inclan g.
- inlay g.
- intercalary g.
- intramedullary g.
- irradiation sterilized g.
- island pedicle g.
- isogenic g.
- jump g.

graft *(continued)*
- Keystone g.
- Krause-Wolfe skin g.
- lyophilized g.
- massive sliding g.
- Matti-Russe g.
- McMaster g.
- mesh g.
- nerve cable g.
- neurovascular pedicle g.
- Nicoll g.
- Ollier-Thiersch skin g.
- onlay g.
- onlay bone g.
- orthotopic g.
- osseous g.
- osteoarticular g.
- osteochondral g.
- osteoperiosteal g.
- pedicle g.
- pedicled bone g.
- peg g.
- periosteal g.
- Phemister g.
- Phemister bone g.
- pinch g.
- quadratus femoris muscle pedicle g.
- Reverdin skin g.
- reversed vein bypass g.
- rib g.
- Robinson horseshoe g.
- Russe g.
- Ryerson g.
- segmental g.
- semitendinosus g.
- skin g.
- sliding inlay g.
- Soto-Hall g.
- spline-type bone g.
- split-thickness skin g.
- Stent g.
- strut g.
- tendon g.
- g. tensioning
- tumbler g.
- wedge g.
- Wilson g.

graft *(continued)*
  Wolfe skin g.
  xenogeneic g.

graft·ing
  bone g.
  nonvascularized bone g.
  vascularized bone g.

Graft Rack

Gra·ham
  G. nerve hook

Gram
  G. stain

Gram·ko
  Buck-G. pollicization

Grand
  Edgarton-G. thumb adduction

gran·u·la·tion

gran·ule
  Kölliker's interstitial g's

gran·u·lo·ma *pl.* gran·u·lo·mas, gran·u·lo·ma·ta
  eosinophilic g.
  giant cell reparative g.
  Mignon's eosinophilic g.
  reticulohistiocytic g.
  rheumatic g's

Grash·ey
  G. view

grasp·er
  suture g.

Graves
  G. scapula

Gray·son
  G. ligament

Grebe
  G. syndrome

Green
  Fried and G. procedure
  G. procedure

Green *(continued)*
  Grice-G. procedure
  Reverdin-G. procedure

Green·field
  Sutherland-G. osteotomy

Greig
  G. cephalopolysyndactyly syndrome

Grice
  G. procedure
  G.-Green procedure

Grif·fin
  Boyd and G. classification (for trochanteric fractures of the femur)

Grif·fith
  G. criterion (for mechanical failure)
  Ma and G. procedure

grip
  hook g.
  power g.
  precision g.

Grip·per Plus ac·e·tab·u·lar cup

Gris·ti·na
  G. and Webb prosthesis

Grit·ti
  G's amputation
  G's operation

grom·met
  titanium g.

groove
  biceps g.
  bicipital g. of humerus
  bicipital g., lateral
  bicipital g., medial
  bicipital g., radial
  bicipital g., ulnar
  costal g.
  interosseous g. of calcaneus

groove *(continued)*
    intertubercular g. of hu-
      merus
    musculospiral g.
    obturator g.
    paraglenoid g's of hip bone
    preauricular g's of ilium
    radial g.
    g. for radial nerve
    Sibson's g.
    spiral g.
    subclavian g.
    subcostal g.
    supra-acetabular g.
    g. for tibialis posticus
      muscle
    ulnar g.
    g. of ulnar nerve
    vertebral g.

Gross
    G.-Kemph nail

Groves
    G. opponensplasty
    Hey-G. procedure
    Hey-G. shelf procedure
    Hey-G.-Kirk graft

Gru·ber
    G's fossa
    G's syndrome
    Meckel-G. syndrome

Gru·ca
    G. procedure

GSB el·bow pros·the·sis

Gschwend
    G., Scheier, and Bahler el-
      bow prosthesis

GTT
    glucose tolerance test

guard·ing
    muscle g.

Guepar ful·ly con·strained de·
vice

Guepar knee pros·the·sis

guide
    bulb-tipped g.
    bulb-tipped reaming g.
    drill g.
    Fischer g.
    Hoffman drill g.
    Mitek drill g.
    nail driving g.
    reaming g.

guide·wire

Guil·lain
    G.-Barré syndrome

Guil·land
    G. sign

Guis·ti·lo
    G. classification (for open
      fractures)

Gun·ston
    G. unconstrained device
    G.-Hult unicompartmental
      device

Gun·ter·berg
    Stener and G. procedure

Gurd
    Mumford-G. procedure

Gus·tui·lo
    G. unconstrained device

gut·ta-per·cha

gut·ter
    lateral g.
    medial g.
    sacral g.

Gu·yon
    G's amputation
    G's canal
    loge de G.
    G's operation

Gyn·o·gen

HA
  hydroxyapatite

Haas
  H. osteotomy
  His-H. procedure

Hack·en·thall
  H. nail

Had·dad
  H.-Riordan arthrodesis

Ha·gie
  H. pin

Hag·lund
  H. deformity
  H's disease

Hag·ner
  H's disease

Haj·du
  H.-Cheney syndrome

Hal·de·man
  H. graft

Ha·le·nol

Hal·i·fax
  H. interlaminar clamp

ha·lis·te·re·sis
  h. cerea

ha·lis·te·ret·ic

Hall
  Pallister-H. syndrome
  Soto-H. graft
  Soto-H. sign

Hal·ler·mann
  H.-Streiff syndrome

hal·lu·cal

hal·lux *pl.* hal·lu·ces
  h. abductus
  h. adductus

hal·lux *(continued)*
  h. dolorosus
  h. extensus
  h. flexus
  h. malleus
  h. rigidus
  h. tortus
  h. valgus
  h. varus

ha·lo
  h. cast
  h. pin
  h. vest

ha·los·te·re·sis

Hal·sted
  H's suture

hal·ter
  cervical h.

Hal·tran

ham·ar·thri·tis

Ha·mas
  H. prosthesis

ham·ate

ha·ma·tum

Ham·il·ton
  H. test

ham·mer
  slap h.
  sliding h.

Ham·mer·schlag
  H's test

ham·mer·toe

Ham·mon
  H. procedure

ham·string
  inner h.
  outer h.

ham·u·lus *pl.* ham·u·li
  h. of hamate bone
  h. ossis hamati

Han·cock
  H's amputation
  H's operation

Hand
  H.-Schüller-Christian disease

hand
  ape h.
  claw h.
  club h.
  flat h.
  frozen h.
  mechanical h.
  mirror h's
  monkey h.
  myelopathy h.
  opera-glass h.
  skeleton h.
  trench h.
  windswept h.
  writing h.

hand chuck

han·dle
  knife h.
  scalpel h.

Han·sen
  H.-Street driver-extractor
  H.-Street nail
  Lauge-H. classification (for ankle fracture)
  Winquist-H. classification (for comminution of femoral fractures)

HAP
  hydroxyapatite

hard·en·ing
  work h.

Hare
  H. traction

Hark
  H. procedure

Har·ley
  Stewart and H. arthrodesis

Har·mon
  H. procedure

har·ness
  A/C (acromioclavicular) h.
  figure 8 h.
  Pavlik h.
  shoulder h.

Har·ri
  H.-Luque technique

Har·ring·ton
  H's classification
  H. distractor
  H. hook clamp
  H. instrumentation
  H. rod
  H. rod fusion
  H. spinal elevator
  Kostuik-H. system

Har·ris
  H. center-cutting reamer
  H. hip score
  H. line
  H. mat
  H. nail
  H. Precoat Plus Prosthesis
  H. total hip replacement
  H.-Beath procedure
  H.-Galante Porous-Coated Hip System
  H.-Galante total hip replacement
  Salter-H. classification
  Salter-H. fracture

Har·ri·son
  H.-Beath differential pressure mat

Har·ti·gan
  H's foramen

har·vest
     graft h.

har·vest·ing
     graft h.

Hass·man
     H., Brunn, and Neer pro-
          cedure

Has·tings
     H. total hip replacement

Hau·ser
     H. procedure
     H. transplant

haus·trum *pl.* haus·tra

ha·ver·sian canal

Haw·kins
     H. sign

Hay
     H.-Wells syndrome

Hay·garth
     H's nodes
     H's nodosities

Hb
     hemoglobin

HB-Ag
     hepatitis B antigen

HB$_s$Ag
     hepatitis B surface anti-
          gen

HBFG
     heparin-binding fibroblast
          growth factor

Hc
     hematocrit

Hct
     hematocrit

HD
     hip disarticulation

HDF
     high dry field

HD-2 Hip

HDR
     Harrington distraction rod

HD-2 to·tal hip re·place·ment

Head
     Mallory-H. Hip
     Mallory-H. prosthesis

head
     articular h.
     h. of astragalus
     coronoid h. of pronator
          teres muscle
     deep h. of flexor pollicis
          brevis
     deep h. of triceps brachii
          muscle
     deep h. of triceps extensor
          cubiti muscle
     h. of femur
     femoral h.
     h. of fibula
     first h. of triceps brachii
          muscle
     first h. of triceps extensor
          cubiti muscle
     great h. of adductor hallu-
          cis muscle
     great h. of triceps brachii
          muscle
     great h. of triceps extensor
          cubiti muscle
     great h. of triceps femoris
          muscle
     humeral h. of flexor carpi
          ulnaris muscle
     humeral h. of flexor digito-
          rum sublimis muscle
     humeral h. of pronator
          teres muscle
     humeroulnar h. of flexor
          digitorum superficialis
          muscle
     h. of humerus
     lateral h. of gastrocnemius
          muscle

head *(continued)*

   lateral h. of triceps brachii muscle

   lateral h. of triceps extensor cubiti muscle

   little h. of humerus

   long h. of adductor hallucis muscle

   long h. of adductor triceps muscle

   long h. of biceps brachii muscle

   long h. of biceps femoris muscle

   long h. of biceps flexor cruris muscle

   long h. of biceps flexor cubiti muscle

   long h. of triceps brachii muscle

   long h. of triceps extensor cubiti muscle

   long h. of triceps femoris muscle

   medial h. of biceps brachii muscle

   medial h. of biceps flexor cubiti muscle

   medial h. of gastrocnemius muscle

   medial h. of triceps brachii muscle

   medial h. of triceps extensor cubiti muscle

   h. of metacarpal

   h. of metatarsal

   middle h. of triceps brachii muscle

   middle h. of triceps extensor cubiti muscle

   h. of muscle

   oblique h. of adductor hallucis muscle

   oblique h. of adductor pollicis muscle

   h. of phalanx of fingers

   h. of phalanx of toes

head *(continued)*

   plantar h. of flexor digitorum pedis longus muscle

   quadrate h. of flexor digitorum pedis longus muscle

   radial h.

   radial h. of flexor digitorum sublimis muscle

   radial h. of flexor digitorum superficialis muscle

   radial h. of humerus

   h. of radius

   h. of rib

   scapular h. of triceps brachii muscle

   scapular h. of triceps extensor cubiti muscle

   second h. of triceps brachii muscle

   short h. of biceps brachii muscle

   short h. of biceps femoris muscle

   short h. of biceps flexor cruris muscle

   short h. of biceps flexor cubiti muscle

   short h. of coracoradialis muscle

   short h. of triceps brachii muscle

   short h. of triceps extensor cubiti muscle

   short h. of triceps femoris muscle

   superficial h. of flexor pollicis brevis

   h. of talus

   transverse h. of adductor hallucis muscle

   transverse h. of adductor pollicis muscle

   h. of ulna

   ulnar h. of flexor carpi ulnaris muscle

   ulnar h. of pronator teres muscle

head·lamp
    fiberoptic h.
    halogen h.

head·rest
    Mayfield pin-holder h.

heal·ing
    fracture h.

Heb·er·den
    H's nodes
    H's rheumatism
    H's signs

he·bos·te·ot·o·my

Hecht
    H. syndrome

heel
    black-dot h.
    gonorrheal h.
    painful h.
    policeman's h.
    prominent h.
    h. strike
    Thomas h.
    torque h.
    walking h.

Hef·fing·ton
    H. frame

Hei·fetz
    H. procedure

height
    patellar h.

Hei·ple
    Marcus, Balourdas, H. ar-
      throdesis

Hel·bing
    H's sign

he·lo·ma
    h. durum

hem·an·gio·blas·to·ma

hem·an·gio·en·do·the·li·o·
ma

hem·an·gi·o·ma

hem·an·gio·peri·cy·to·ma

hem·an·gio·sar·co·ma

hem·a·poph·y·sis

hem·ar·thros

hem·ar·thro·sis

he·ma·to·crit

hem·a·to·ma *pl.* hem·a·
tomas
    intramuscular h.

he·ma·to·my·e·lia

hem·a·tor·rha·chis

hem·a·tos·te·on

he·ma·tox·y·lin

hemi·ar·thro·plas·ty
    bipolar h.

hemi·ar·thro·sis

hemi·cen·trum

hemi·lam·i·nec·to·my

hemi·lam·i·not·o·my

hemi·me·lia
    complete paraxial h.
    dysplasia epiphysealis h.
    incomplete paraxial h
    paraxial h.
    partial h.

hemi·pel·vec·to·my
    internal h.

hemi·phal·an·gec·to·my

hemi·ple·gia
    double h.

hemi·ple·gic

hemi·sa·cral·iza·tion

hemi·teno·de·sis

hemi·ver·te·bra

he·mo·chro·ma·to·sis

he·mo·glo·bin
    mean corpuscular h. con-
        centration

he·mo·phil·ia

he·mor·rhage

he·mo·sid·er·in

he·mo·stat
    Kelly h.

Hench
    H.-Rosenberg syndrome

Hen·der·son
    Charnley and H. arthro-
        desis
    H. arthrodesis
    H. graft
    H. lag screw
    H.-Jones chondromatosis

Hen·le
    crural canal of H.
    inferior ligament of neck
        of rib of H.
    H's ligament
    scapular tuberosity of H.
    superior tubercle of H.
    trapezoid bone of H.

Hen·ry
    H. graft
    H. and Wrisberg ligament

Hen·schke
    H.-Mauch prosthesis

Hen·sen
    H's disk
    H's line
    H's plane

Her·bert
    H. bone screw
    H's classification (for
        scaphoid fractures)
    H. fully constrained device
    H. jig
    H. screw
    H. unconstrained device

Her·mods·son
    H. fracture

Hern·don
    Borden, Spencer, and H.
        osteotomy
    H.-Heyman procedure
    Heyman-H. procedure

her·nia
    Birkett's h.
    synovial h.

her·ni·at·ed

her·ni·a·tion
    disk h.
    foraminal disk h.
    intradural disk h.
    intraosseous h.
    intraspongy nuclear h.
    lateral disk h.
    lumbar disk h.
    painful fat h.
    recurrent lumbar disk h.

Her·zog
    H's curve

Hes·sel
    H./Nystrom pin

het·ero·graft

het·ero-os·teo·plas·ty

Heu·ter
    H. line

Hex·a·brix

Hex-Fix ex·ter·nal fix·a·tion
    sys·tem

Hey
    H's amputation
    H's internal derangement
    H's operation
    H's procedure
    H's saw
    H.-Groves shelf procedure
    H.-Groves-Kirk graft

Hey·man
    Herndon-H. procedure
    H.-Herndon procedure

HFFTTA
    hypermobile flat foot with
    tight tendo Achillis

Hgb
    hemoglobin

H&H
    hemoglobin and hemato-
    crit

HHS
    Harris hip score

hi·a·tus
    adductor h.
    h. adductorius
    h. finalis sacralis
    h. intermedius lumbosa-
    cralis
    h. interosseus
    h. lumbosacralis
    sacral h.
    h. sacralis
    saphenous h.
    h. saphenus
    h. tendineus
    h. totalis sacralis

Hibbs
    H. arthrodesis
    H. gouge
    H. operation
    H. osteotome
    H. procedure
    H. retractor
    H. spinal fusion

HID
    herniated intervertebral
    disk

Hil·gen·rein·er
    H. angle

Hill
    Baker and H. osteotomy
    H.-Sachs fracture

Hill *(continued)*
    H.-Sachs lesion

hind·foot

hinge
    elbow h.
    flail-elbow h.
    flexible h.
    internal positive locking h.
    multiple-action h.
    outside locking h.
    single-pivot h.
    sliding action step-up h.
    stump-activated locking h.
    suspension polycentric h.

Hip
    hip amputation

hip
    ankylosed h.
    HD-2 H.
    hybrid h.
    Indiana Conservative H.
    Lubinus h.
    Mallory-Head H.
    observation h.
    PCA Porous-Coated H.
    h. pointer
    Precision H.
    Precision Osteoblock H.
    primary h.
    silent h.
    snapping h.

Hirsch·berg
    H. sign

His
    H.-Haas procedure

his·tio·cyte

his·tio·cy·to·ma
    benign fibrous h.
    fibrous h.
    malignant h.
    malignant fibrous h.

his·tio·di·no·hy·droxy·mero·
des·mo·sine

his·tio-ir·ri·ta·tive

his·to·com·pa·ti·bil·i·ty

His·to·plas·ma

HIT
    hypertrophic infiltrative
        tendinitis

Hitch·cock
    H. procedure

HKAFO
    hip-knee-ankle-foot or-
        thosis

HNP
    herniated nucleus pulpo-
        sus

HO
    hip orthosis

Hoag·lund
    H. graft

Hobb
    H. view

Hodg·en
    H. splint

Hodg·kin
    H's disease
    H. tumor

Hodg·son
    H. procedure
    H. rongeur

Hof·fa
    H's disease
    H. fat

Hof·fer
    H. procedure

Hoff·man
    H. drill guide
    H. fixation device
    H.-Vital fixation device

Hoff·mann
    H. sign

Hohl
    H. fracture

Hoh·mann
    H. procedure
    H. retractor

Hoke
    H. procedure

hol·ar·thri·tis

Hol·den
    H's line

hold·er
    arthroscopic shoulder h.
    needle h.
    Steinmann pin h.
    tibial track h.

Hol·lis·ter
    Levy-H. syndrome

hol·low-back

Hol·scher
    H. root retractor

Holt
    H.-Oram syndrome

Homans
    H. sign

ho·meo-os·teo·plas·ty

ho·mo·graft

Hon·vol

hood
    dorsal h.

hook
    Anatomic h.
    Anatomic II h.
    APRL (Army Prosthetics
        Research Laboratory) h.
    bone h.
    bony h.
    gaff h.
    Graham nerve h.
    hamate h.
    Moe sacral h's

hook *(continued)*
    nerve h.
    suture h.
    Trautman Locktite h.

Hoo·ver
    H. test

Hor·mo·gen De·pot

hor·mone
    growth h. (GH)
    growth hormone release
      inhibiting h. (GH-RIH)
    human (pituitary) growth
      h. (hGH)
    parathyroid h.
    placental growth h.
    thyroid-stimulating h.
      (TSH)

horn
    coccygeal h.
    inferior h. of falciform
      margin
    posterior h. of lateral ven-
      tricle
    posterior h. of spinal cord
    retained posterior h.
    sacral h.
    superior h. of falciform
      margin

Ho·ros
    Marcove, Lewis, and H.
      procedure

Hor·witz
    H. and Adams arthrodesis

Hos·pi·tal for Spe·cial Sur·
    gery Hip Rat·ing Scale

Hos·pi·tal for Spe·cial Sur·
    gery Knee Rat·ing Scale

Ho·va·ni·an
    H. procedure

How·ard
    Copeland and H. proce-
      dure
    Kenney-H. splint

Ho·worth
    H. reduction

Howse
    H. total hip replacement

How·ship
    H. lacuna

HPF
    high-power field

HS25

HSS semi·con·strained de·
    vice

Hu·ber
    H. opponensplasty

Huck·step
    H. nail

Hud·son
    H. brace

Hue·ter
    H's line
    H. sign

Hughes
    Sukhtian-H. fixation de·
      vice

Hugh·ston
    Darrach-H.-Milch fracture
    Dimon and H. procedure
    H. jerk test
    H. procedure
    H. test
    H. view
    H. and Jacobson procedure

Hult
    Gunston-H. unicompart-
      mental device

hu·mer·al

hu·meri

hu·mero·ra·di·al

hu·mero·scap·u·lar

hu·mero·ul·nar

hu·mer·us *pl.* hu·meri
    condylar h.
    fracture of h.
    head of h.
    supracondylar h.
    h. varus

hump
    dowager's h.

hump·back

Hum·phrey
    inferior tubercle of H.
    superior tubercle of H.

Hum·phry
    H's ligament

hunch·back

Hü·ner·mann
    chondrodysplasia punc-
      tata, Conradi-H. type

Hunt·er
    H. active tendon implant
    H's canal
    H. passive tendon implant
    H. rod
    H's syndrome
    inferior opening of H's ca-
      nal

Hunt·ing·ton
    H. graft
    H. sign

Hur·ler
    H. syndrome
    H.-Scheie compound syn-
      drome

Hutch·ins
    Anderson and H. proce-
      dure

hy·al·uron·ic acid

hy·al·uron·i·dase

Hyb·bi·nette
    Eden-H. procedure

hy·drar·thro·di·al

hy·drar·thro·sis
    intermittent h.

hy·drath·ro·sis

hy·drops
    h. articuli

hy·droxy·ap·a·tite

hy·droxy·chlo·ro·quine
    h. sulfate

hy·drox·yl·ap·a·tite
    H. McCutchen Total Hip
      System

hy·drox·y·ly·sine

hy·drox·y·ly·sin·o·nor·leu·
cine

p-hy·droxy·mer·cu·ri·ben·zo·
ate

hy·droxy·pro·line

hy·gro·ma *pl.* hy·gro·mas,
   hy·gro·ma·ta
    h. praepatellare

hyp·al·ge·sia

Hy·paque-76

Hy·paque-M

Hy·paque Me·glu·mine

Hy·paque Oral

Hy·paque So·di·um

hy·per·al·ge·sia

hy·per·cho·les·ter·emia

hy·per·chon·dro·pla·sia

hy·per·es·the·sia

hy·per·ex·ten·sion

hy·per·flex·ion

hy·per·gly·ce·mia

hy·per·lor·do·sis

hy·per·mo·bil·i·ty
    segmental h.

hy·per·os·te·og·e·ny

hy·per·os·to·sis
  ankylosing h.
  ankylosing spinal h.
  h. corticalis deformans juvenilis
  h. corticalis generalisata
  diffuse idiopathic sclerosing h.
  diffuse idiopathic skeletal h.
  flowing h.
  infantile cortical h.
  senile ankylosing h. of spine

hy·per·os·tot·ic

hy·per·para·thy·roid·ism

hy·per·phos·pha·ta·se·mia
  chronic congenital idiopathic h.
  h. tarda

hy·per·pla·sia
  epiphyseal h.

hy·per·plas·tic

hy·per·spon·gi·o·sis

hy·per·telo·rism

hy·per·ten·sion

hy·per·thy·roid·ism

hy·per·to·nia

hy·per·ton·ic

hy·per·tro·phia

hy·per·troph·ic

hy·per·tro·phy
  pseudomuscular h.

hy·per·vi·ta·min·o·sis
  h. D

hy·po·chon·dro·pla·sia

hy·po·con·dy·lar

hy·po·es·the·sia

hy·po·gly·ce·mia

hy·po·ky·pho·sis

hy·po·nych·i·um

hy·po·para·thy·roid·ism

hy·po·phos·pha·ta·sia

hy·po·pla·sia
  cartilage-hair h.

hy·po·po·ro·sis

hyp·os·to·sis

hy·po·telo·rism

hy·po·ten·sion

hy·poth·e·nar

hy·poth·e·sis
  sliding-filament h.

hy·po·thy·roid·ism

hy·po·ton·ic

hy·po·vo·le·mia

hy·pox·ia

hys·te·re·sis

I
    intercalary (congenital absence of limb)

IAT
    intraoperative autologous transfusion

Ib·ren

Ibu·med

Ibu·prin

Ibu·pro-600

ibu·pro·fen

Ibu·prohm

Ibu-Tab

Ibu·tex

ICB
    intercostal nerve block

ICLH an·kle pros·the·sis

ICLH el·bow pros·the·sis

ICLH un·con·strained de·vice

I&D
    incision and drainage

IDE
    investigational device exemption

id·io·path·ic

IDK
    idiopathic derangement of the knee

Ifen

Iku·ta
    I. fixation device

ILCH dou·ble cup ar·thro·plas·ty

Il·feld
    I. splint

il·ia

il·i·ac

il·io·coc·cyg·e·al

il·io·cos·tal

il·io·fem·or·al

il·io·pso·as

il·io·sa·cral

il·io·sci·at·ic

il·io·spi·nal

il·io·tib·i·al

il·io·tro·chan·ter·ic

il·i·um *pl.* il·ia

Ili·za·rov
    I. fixation device

im·age
    T1 weighted i.
    T2 weighted i.

imag·ing
    magnetic resonance i. (MRI)

im·bal·ance
    musculotendinous i.

im·bri·ca·tion

imi·pen·em
    i. and cilastatin

im·mo·bil·iza·tion
    cast i.

im·mo·bi·lize

im·mu·no·elec·tro·pho·re·sis

im·mu·no·sup·pres·sion

im·pac·tion
   atlantoaxial i.

im·pac·tor
   Cloward i.
   extractor-i.
   i.-extractor

im·pac·tor-ex·trac·tor

IMP-Ca·pel·lo slim·line ab·
   duc·tion pil·low

im·pinge·ment
   cervicomedullary i.
   cord i.
   root i.
   spinal i.

im·plant
   concave condylar i.
   convex condylar i.
   custom i.
   Eaton trapezium i.
   hinged i.
   Hunter active tendon i.
   Hunter passive tendon i.
   lunate i.
   metal i.
   neck-head i.
   Niebauer i.
   orthopedic i.
   Osteonics-HA femoral i.
   scaphoid i.
   stemmed i.
   Swanson i.
   Swanson carpal scaphoid i.
   tibial i.
   transcortical i.
   trapezium i.

im·plan·ta·tion
   periosteal i.

im·pres·sio pl. im·pres·si·o·
   nes
      i. ligamenti costoclavicu-
         laris

im·pres·sion
   basilar i.

im·pres·sion (continued)
   i. of costoclavicular liga-
      ment
   deltoid i. of humerus
   rhomboid i. of clavicle

im·pulse

Im·u·ran

in·car·cer·a·tion
   nail i.

in·ci·sion
   deltoid-splitting i.
   i. and drainage
   Kessel i.
   lateral parapatellar i.
   medial parapatellar i.
   pararectus i.
   Wagner i.

in·ci·su·ra pl. in·ci·su·rae
   i. acetabuli
   i. clavicularis sterni
   incisurae costales sterni
   i. fibularis tibiae
   i. ischiadica major
   i. ischiadica minor
   i. ischialis major
   i. ischialis minor
   i. jugularis sterni
   i. peronea tibiae
   i. radialis ulnae
   i. scapulae
   i. semilunaris tibiae
   i. semilunaris ulnae
   i. trochlearis ulnae
   i. ulnaris radii
   i. vertebralis inferior
   i. vertebralis superior

in·ci·sure
   i. of acetabulum
   i. of calcaneus
   clavicular i. of sternum
   costal i's of sternum
   cotyloid i.
   fibular i. of tibia
   humeral i. of ulna
   iliac i., lesser

in·ci·sure *(continued)*
    interclavicular i.
    ischial i., greater
    ischial i., lesser
    i. of ischium, greater
    i. of ischium, lesser
    jugular i. of sternum
    lateral i. of sternum
    obturator i. of pubic bone
    patellar i. of femur
    peroneal i. of tibia
    popliteal i.
    radial i. of ulna
    i. of scapula
    semilunar i.
    semilunar i., greater, of ulna
    semilunar i., lesser, of ulna
    semilunar i. of radius
    semilunar i. of scapula
    semilunar i. of sternum
    semilunar i. of sternum, superior
    semilunar i. of tibia
    semilunar i. of ulna
    sigmoid i. of ulna
    sternal i.
    suprascapular i.
    i. of talus
    thoracic i.
    trochlear i. of ulna
    ulnar i. of radius
    vertebral i., greater
    vertebral i., inferior
    vertebral i., lesser
    vertebral i., superior

In·clan
    I. graft
    I.-Ober procedure

in·cli·na·tio *pl.* in·cli·na·ti·o·nes
    i. pelvis

in·cli·na·tion
    pelvic i.
    i. of pelvis

in·cli·na·tion *(continued)*
    sacral i.

in·cline
    i. of pelvis
    pelvic i.

in·cli·nom·e·ter

in·con·gru·ence
    patellofemoral i.

in·con·gru·ent

in·cor·po·ra·tion

In·da·meth

in·dex *pl.* in·dex·es, in·di·ces
    ankle-arm i.
    Blackburne and Peel i.
    cortical i.
    mean cortical i.
    Schober's i.
    Singh i.
    valgus i.

In·di·a·na Con·ser·va·tive Hip

In·di·a·na con·ser·va·tive hip ar·thro·plas·ty

In·di·a·na con·ser·va·tive pros·the·sis

In·di·a·na con·ser·va·tive re·sur·fac·ing pro·ce·dure

in·di·ca·tor

In·do·cid

In·do·cin

in·do·meth·a·cin

in·du·ra·tion
    Froriep's i.

in·er·tia

in·farct
    bone i.

in·farc·tion
    bone i.
    Freiberg's i.

in·fec·tion
　　disk space i.
　　Melanie i.
　　pin tract i.
　　spinal i.

in·fe·ri·or

in·fil·tra·tion

in·flam·ma·tion

in·flam·ma·to·ry

in·fra·cot·y·loid

in·frac·tion
　　Freiberg's i.

in·fra·gle·noid

in·fra·pa·tel·lar

in·fra·spi·na·tus

in·fra·spi·nous

in·fun·dib·u·lum *pl.* in·fun·dib·u·la
　　crural i.
　　i. crurale

in·fu·sion

In·gram
　　I. osteotomy
　　I. procedure

in·growth
　　bone i.

in·gui·nal

in·jec·tion
　　trigger point i.

in·ju·ry
　　abduction i.
　　adduction i.
　　factitious i.
　　flexion-compression i.
　　flexion-distraction i.
　　Goyrand's i.
　　overuse i.
　　shear i.
　　skier's i.

in·ju·ry *(continued)*
　　spinal cord i.
　　sports-related i.
　　stress i.
　　torsional i.

in·let
　　pelvic i.

ino·chon·dri·tis

ino·myo·si·tis

ino·phrag·ma

in·os·to·sis

ino·tag·ma

in·ot·ro·pism

In·sall
　　I.-Burstein II modular
　　　　knee system
　　I.-Burstein prosthesis
　　I.-Burstein semicon-
　　　　strained device
　　I.-Salvati ratio

in·sco·li·o·sis
　　fixed curve i.

in·scrip·tio *pl.* in·scrip·ti·o·nes
　　i. tendinea
　　inscriptiones tendineae
　　　　musculi recti abdominis

in·scrip·tion
　　tendinous i.
　　tendinous i's of rectus ab-
　　　　dominis muscle

in·sert
　　lateral i.
　　New York University i.
　　NYU i.
　　silicone gel socket i.
　　soft socket i.
　　sole i.
　　UC-BL i.

in·sert·er
　　Massie i.

in·sert·er *(continued)*
    staple i.

in·sert·er-ex·trac·tor
    compression i.-e.

in si·tu

in·sta·bil·i·ty
    angular i.
    anterior i.
    anterior glenohumeral i.
    anterior-posterior i.
    anteromedial i.
    anteroposterior i.
    axial i.
    axial rotational i.
    carpal i.
    clinical i.
    dorsiflexed intercalated
      segmental i. (DISI)
    inversion-eversion i.
    lateral i.
    lumbar i.
    medial i.
    multidirectional i.
    patellofemoral i.
    posterior i.
    posterolateral i.
    posteromedial i.
    retrolisthetic i.
    rotational i.
    segmental i.
    shoulder i.
    spinal i.
    translational i.
    varus/valgus i.
    volarflexed intercalated
      scapholunate i.

In·stan·tine

in·step

in·stru·ment
    cutdown i's

in·stru·men·ta·tion
    Anspach 65K i.
    Cloward i.
    Cotrel-Dubousset i.

in·stru·men·ta·tion
  (continued)
    Dwyer i.
    Ellipticut i.
    Harrington i.
    lumbar i.
    Luque i.
    Luque/Galveston i.
    modular i.
    Modular System I.
    rod-sleeve i.
    Zielke i.

in·suf·fi·cien·cy
    active i.
    arterial i.
    muscular i.
    venous i.

In·te·gral hip re·place·ment
  sys·tem

In·te·grat·ed Shape Imag·ing
  Sys·tem

in·ter·ac·ces·so·ry

in·ter·ar·tic·u·lar

in·ter·ca·lary

in·ter·car·pal

in·ter·coc·cyg·e·al

in·ter·con·dy·lar

in·ter·con·dy·loid

in·ter·con·dy·lous

in·ter·di·aph·y·se·al

in·ter·dig·it

in·ter·dig·i·tal

in·ter·face
    bone-prosthesis i.

in·ter·frag·men·tary

in·ter·lam·i·nar

in·ter·mal·le·o·lar

in·ter·meta·car·pal

in·ter·meta·tar·sal

in·ter·os·se·ous
    dorsal i.
    volar i.

in·ter·pe·dic·u·late

in·ter·pha·lan·ge·al

in·ter·scap·u·lo·tho·rac·ic

in·ter·sec·tio *pl.* in·ter·sec·
ti·o·nes
    i. tendinea
    intersectiones tendineae
      musculi recti abdominis

in·ter·sec·tion
    tendinous i.

in·ter·space

in·ter·spi·nal

in·ter·spi·nous

in·ter·ster·nal

in·ter·sti·tial

in·ter·tar·sal

in·ter·ten·di·nous

in·ter·trans·verse

in·ter·tro·chan·ter·ic

in·ter·val
    atlantodens i. (ADI)

in·ter·ver·te·bral

in·ti·ma

in·tra·ar·tic·u·lar

in·tra·bur·sal

In·tra·bu·ta·zone

in·tra·cap·su·lar

in·tra·car·pal

in·tra·car·ti·lag·i·nous

in·tra·chon·dral

in·tra·chon·dri·al

in·tra·cos·tal

in·tra·cru·re·us

in·tra·dis·kal

in·tra·ep·i·phys·e·al

in·tra·fu·sal

in·tra·lig·a·men·tous

in·tra·med·ul·lary

in·tra·os·se·ous

in·tra·os·te·al

in·tra·sa·cral

in·tra·spi·nous

in·tra·ster·nal

in·tra·syno·vi·al

in·tra·tar·sal

in·tra·the·nar

in·tro·i·tus *pl.* in·tro·i·tus
    i. pelvis

in·tu·ba·tion

in·vag·i·na·tion
    basilar i.

in·ver·sion
    ankle stress i.

in vi·tro

in vi·vo

in·vo·lu·crum *pl.* in·vo·lu·
cra

In·yo
    I. nail

io·hex·ol

Io·nes·cu
    Veleanu, Rosianu, and I.
      procedure

io·thal·a·mate
    i. meglumine

Io·wa Hip Rat·ing Scale

Io·wa to·tal hip re·place·
    ment

iox·a·glate

IP
    interphalangeal

IP ex·ten·sion as·sist

IPSF
    immediate postsurgical fit-
        ting

ip·si·lat·er·al

IRM spi·ral or·tho·sis

ir·ri·ga·tion
    closed suction i.

ir·ri·ta·bil·i·ty
    residual nerve root i.

Ir·win
    I. osteotomy

is·che·mia
    brachiocephalic i.
    muscle i.
    Volkmann's i.

is·chia

is·chi·al·gia

is·chi·ec·to·my

is·chio·cap·su·lar

is·chio·coc·cyg·e·al

is·chio·dyn·ia

is·chio·fem·o·ral

is·chio·fib·u·lar

is·chio·he·bot·o·my

is·chio·ni·tis

is·chio·pu·bic

is·chio·pu·bi·ot·o·my

is·chio·sa·cral

is·chio·ver·te·bral

is·chi·um *pl.* is·chia

Ishi·zu·ki
    I. elbow prosthesis

ISIS
    Integrated Shape Imaging
        System

is·land
    bone i.

iso·an·ti·body

iso·graft

iso·ki·net·ic

ISOLA Spi·nal Sys·tem

Isom·e·ter

isom·e·try

Iso·tac

iso·ton·ic

iso·trop·ic

Is·rael
    I. retractor

ISSLS
    International Society for
        the Study of the Lumbar
        Spine

isth·mus *pl.* is·thmi

ith·y·cy·phos

ith·y·lor·do·sis

ith·yo·ky·pho·sis

IV-type ba·sic frame

J
  joint

Ja·bou·lay
  J's amputation
  J's operation

Jac·coud
  J's sign

jack·et
  body j.
  Lexan j.
  Minerva j.
  plaster of Paris j.
  Prenyl j.
  Wilmington j.

jack·so·ni·an ep·i·lep·sy

Ja·cob
  J. shift test

Ja·cobs
  J. chuck
  Wilson and J. procedure

Ja·cob·son
  Hughston and J. procedure

Ja·cov·sky
  J's projection

Jaf·fe
  J's disease

Jaf·fee
  J. total hip replacement

Ja·mar
  J. dynamometer

Ja·nec·ki
  J. and Nelson procedure

Jan·sen
  J's disease
  J. test
  metaphyseal chondrodys-
    plasia, J. type

Ja·pas
  J. osteotomy
  J. procedure

Jar·cho
  J.-Levin syndrome

Jean·selme
  J's nodules

Jeb·son
  J.-Taylor hand function
    test

Jef·fer·son
  J. fracture

Jen·a·mi·cin

Jen·dras·sik
  J. maneuver

Jeune
  J. thoracic dystrophy

Jew·ett
  J. brace
  J. driver
  J. nail
  J. orthosis

jig
  cutting j.
  Herbert j.

Jo·bert
  J's fossa

Jo·hans·son
  Sinding-Larsen-J. disease

John C. Wil·son
  J.C.W. arthrodesis

John·ell
  Redlund-J. method

joint
  A/C (acromioclavicular) j.
  acromioclavicular j.
  amphidiarthrodial j.

joint *(continued)*
- ankle j.
- arthrodial j.
- atlantoaxial j.
- atlantodental j.
- atlanto-occipital j.
- ball-and-socket j.
- basal j.
- biaxial j.
- bicondylar j.
- bilocular j.
- bleeders' j.
- brachiocarpal j.
- brachioradial j.
- brachioulnar j.
- calcaneocuboid j.
- capitular j.
- carpal j's
- carpometacarpal j's
- carpometacarpal j. of thumb
- cartilaginous j.
- Charcot's j.
- Chopart's j.
- Clutton's j.
- coccygeal j.
- cochlear j.
- composite j.
- compound j.
- condylar j.
- condyloid j.
- costocentral j.
- costochondral j's
- costotransverse j.
- costovertebral j's
- coxofemoral j. of Buisson
- cricoarytenoid j.
- Cruveilhier's j.
- cubital j.
- cuboideonavicular j.
- cuneocuboid j.
- cuneometatarsal j.
- cuneonavicular j.
- diarthrodial j.
- j. disease
- distal radioulnar j.
- double-action ankle j.
- dry j.

joint *(continued)*
- elastic knee cage with contoured knee j.
- elbow j.
- ellipsoidal j.
- enarthrodial j.
- facet j's
- false j.
- femoral j.
- femoropatellar j.
- femorotibial j.
- fibrocartilaginous j.
- fibrous j's
- first carpometacarpal j.
- flail j.
- j. fracture
- free-action ankle j.
- freely movable j.
- free-motion ankle j.
- fringe j.
- ginglymoid j.
- glenohumeral j.
- gliding j.
- hemophilic j.
- hinge j.
- hip j.
- humeroradial j.
- humeroulnar j.
- immovable j.
- inferior radioulnar j.
- inferior sternal j.
- inferior tibiofibular j.
- inflammatory j.
- interarticular j's
- intercarpal j's
- interchondral j's
- intercuneiform j's
- intermetacarpal j's
- intermetatarsal j's
- internal derangement of j.
- interphalangeal j's
- interphalangeal j's of fingers
- interphalangeal j's of foot
- interphalangeal j's of hand
- interphalangeal j's of toes
- intertarsal j's
- intervertebral j.

joint *(continued)*
    irritable j.
    knee j.
    lateral atlantoaxial j.
    ligamentous j.
    limited motion ankle j.
    limited-action ankle j.
    Lisfranc's j.
    lumbosacral j.
    j's of Luschka
    Luschka's j.
    mandibular j.
    manubriosternal j.
    medial atlantoaxial j.
    mediocarpal j.
    metacarpophalangeal j's
    metatarsophalangeal j's
    metatarsophalangeal j.
      dislocation
    midcarpal j.
    midtarsal j.
    mixed j.
    movable j.
    multiaxial j.
    neurocentral j.
    orthotic ankle j.
    orthotic knee j.
    patellofemoral j.
    j. of pisiform bone
    pisotriquetral j.
    pivot j.
    plane j.
    polyaxial j.
    proximal radioulnar j.
    radiocarpal j.
    rotary j.
    sacrococcygeal j.
    sacroiliac j.
    saddle j.
    scaphotrapezial j.
    scapuloclavicular j.
    scapulothoracic j.
    sellar j.
    j. separation
    shoulder j.
    simple j.
    slip j.
    spheroidal j.

joint *(continued)*
    spiral j.
    sternoclavicular j.
    sternocostal j's
    j. stiffness
    subtalar j.
    superior radioulnar j.
    superior sternal j.
    superior tibiofibular j.
    Swanson toe j.
    synarthrodial j's
    synovial j.
    talocalcaneonavicular j.
    talocrural j.
    talonavicular j.
    talotibiofibular j.
    tarsal j., transverse
    tarsometatarsal j's
    temporomandibular j.
    temporomaxillary j.
    through j.
    thumb basal j's
    tibiofibular j.
    transverse tarsal j.
    trapeziometacarpal j.
    trapezioscaphoid j.
    trapeziotrapezoid j.
    trochoid j.
    trochoidal j.
    uncovertebral j.
    uniaxial j.
    unilocular j.
    virgin j.
    von Gies j.
    weight-bearing j.
    wrist j.
    xiphisternal j.
    zygapophyseal j's

Jones
    Blundell J. hip osteotomy
    Blundell J. varus osteot-
      omy
    Henderson-J. chondroma-
      tosis
    J. abduction frame
    J. fracture
    J. position

Jones *(continued)*
  J. procedure
  Lam modification of J.
    procedure
  Robert J. bandage
  Watson-J. arthrodesis
  Watson-J. procedure

J.R. Moore
  J.R.M. procedure

JT
  joint

Jts
  joints

Ju·det
  J. femoral head component
  J. total hip replacement

jump·er's knee

junc·tion
  cervicodorsal j.
  cervicothoracic j.
  costochondral j.
  lumbosacral j.
  manubriogladiolar j.
  musculotendinous j.
  occipitoatlantal (OA) j.
  osseous j's

junc·tion *(continued)*
  tendinous j's
  thoracolumbar j.

junc·tu·ra *pl.* junc·tu·rae
  juncturae cartilagineae
  juncturae cinguli membri
    inferioris
  juncturae cinguli membri
    superioris
  juncturae columnae verte-
    bralis, thoracis, et cranii
  juncturae fibrosae
  j. lumbosacralis
  juncturae membri infer-
    ioris liberi
  juncturae membri superi-
    oris liberi
  j. ossium
  juncturae ossium
  j. sacrococcygea
  juncturae synoviales
  juncturae tendinum
  juncturae zygapophyseales

junc·tu·rae

Ju·vara
  J. procedure

jux·ta·po·si·tion

KAFO
  knee-ankle-foot orthosis

Kag·er
  K's triangle

Kam·bin
  K's triangular working
    zone

kan·a·my·cin

Kan·a·vel
  K's sign
  K's triangle

Ka·ne·da
  K. device

Kan·trex

Ka·pel
  K. procedure

Kap·lan
  K's fibers

Kar·kou·sis
  K. and Vezeridis proce-
    dure

Ka·shin
  K.-Beck disease

Kast
  K's syndrome

Ka·to
  K's test

Kau·fer
  K. procedure

Ka·wa·sa·ki
  K. disease

Keen
  K's sign

Kef·let

Kef·lex

Kef·lin

Kef·tab

Kef·ur·ox

Kef·zol

Keio
  Leids-K. ligament

Ke·li·ki·an
  K. tendon transfer

Kel·ler
  K. operation
  K. procedure

Kel·ley
  K. gouge

Kel·ly
  K. clamp
  K. hemostat

ke·loid
  Addison's k.

Kemph
  Gross-K. nail

Ken
  K. driver-extractor
  K. nail
  K. screwdriver
  K. sliding nail

Ken·drick
  K. procedure

Ken·ne·dy
  K. ligament augmentation
    device

Ken·ney
  K.-Howard splint
  intractable plantar k.

ker·a·to·ma *pl.* ker·a·to·
  mas, ker·a·to·ma·ta

ker·a·to·sis *pl.* ker·a·to·ses
    intractable plantar k.

Ker·lix dress·ing

Kern
    K. bone holding forceps

Ker·nig
    K. sign

Kerr
    K. sign

Ker·ri·son
    K. punch
    K. rongeur

Kes·sel
    K. incision

Kes·sler
    K. procedure
    K. prosthesis
    K. suture
    K. tendon repair

Kes·trin Aq·ue·ous

Kes·trone-5

ke·to·pro·fen

Key
    K. arthrodesis
    K. periosteal elevator

Kic·kal·dy
    K. and Willis arthrodesis

Kid·ner
    K. procedure

Kiehn
    K.-Earle-DesPrez proce-
       dure

Kiel
    K. bone

Kien·böck
    K's disease
    K's dislocation

Kil·i·an
    K's line

Kil·li·an
    K. and Teschler-Nicola
       syndrome

kilo·pond

kine·mat·ic

Kine·mat·ic ful·ly con·
    strained de·vice

Kine·mat·ic II semi·con·
    strained de·vice

kine·mat·ics
    joint k.

Kin·e·max Plus To·tal Knee
    Sys·tem

kine·plas·tics

kine·plas·ty

kine·sal·gia

ki·ne·si·al·gia

ki·ne·si·ol·o·gy

ki·net·ics
    joint k.

ki·ne·tron

King
    K. and Steelquist amputa-
       tion
    Reichenheim-K. procedure

kink·ing
    pedicular k.

Kirk
    Hey-Groves-K. graft
    K's amputation

Kir·ner
    K. deformity

Kirsch·ner
    K. wire
    K. wire skeletal traction
    K. wire splint

Kit·tel
    K's treatment

Klapp
  K's creeping treatment

Kleb·si·el·la

Klei·ger
  Tillaux K. fracture

Klein·ert
  K. tendon repair

Klemm
  K.-Schellmann locking
    nail

Klen·zak
  K. orthosis

Kline·fel·ter
  K's syndrome

Kling
  K. arthrodesis
  K. dressing

Klip·pel
  K.-Feil sequence
  K.-Trenaunay-Weber syn-
    drome

knee
  anterior detachment of k.
  back k.
  beat k.
  breaststroker's k.
  Brodie's k.
  congenital dislocation of k.
  disarticulation of k.
  dislocation of k.
  football k.
  fracture of k.
  hamstrung k.
  housemaid's k.
  in k.
  jumper's k.
  knock k.
  locked k.
  Omnifit Total K.
  k. orthosis
  out k.
  k. prosthesis
  rugby k.

knee *(continued)*
  runner's k.
  SCR single compartment
    replacement k.
  septic k.
  k. sprain
  trick k.
  valgus k.
  varus k.
  virgin k.

Knee So·ci·e·ty Knee Score

Kniest
  K. dysplasia

knife
  Bard-Parker k.
  Downing cartilage k.
  Krull acetabular k.
  Liston's k.
  orthopedic k.
  Rosen k.
  Smillie cartilage k.

Knight
  K.-Taylor orthosis

knit·ting

knock-knee

Knodt
  K. distraction
  K. rods
  clove-hitch k.

Knott
  K. test

Knowles
  K. pin

KO
  knee orthosis

Koch
  K.-Mason dressing

Koch·er
  K. approach
  K. clamp
  K. clamp test
  K. fracture

Koch·er *(continued)*
  K's operation

Köh·ler
  K's bone disease
  K's disease
  K's line
  K's second disease

koi·lor·rhach·ic

koi·lo·ster·nia

Köl·li·ker
  column of K.
  K's interstitial granules

Kö·ning
  K's disease

Kon·stram
  K. angle

Kort·zen·born
  K. procedure

Koz·low·ski
  K. spondylometaphyseal
    dysplasia

Kos·tu·ik
  K.-Harrington system

Krac·kow
  K. suture

Kra·mer
  K., Craig, and Noel osteot-
    omy

Krause
  K's line
  K's membrane
  K.-Wolfe skin graft
  posterior costotransverse
    ligament of K.

Kru·ken·berg
  K. procedure

Krull
  K. acetabular knife

KT-1000 ar·throm·e·ter

Ku·do
  K. elbow prosthesis

Küm·mell
  K's disease
  K's spondylitis

Künt·scher
  K. awl
  K. driver
  K. extractor
  K. modified arthrodesis
  K. nail
  K. ossimeter
  K. rod

Ku·ro·sa·ka
  K. screw

Kus·ko·kwim
  K. disease

Kut·ler
  K. amputation
  K. flap

K-wire fix·a·tion

K-wire skel·e·tal trac·tion

kyl·lo·sis

ky·pho·re·duc·tion

ky·phos

ky·pho·sco·li·o·sis

ky·pho·sis
  cervical k.
  k. dorsalis juvenilis
  juvenile k.
  lumbar k.
  lumbosacral k.
  post-traumatic k.
  Scheuermann's k.

ky·phot·ic

kyr·tor·rhach·ic

la·bi·um *pl.* la·bia
l. externum cristae iliacae
l. internum cristae iliacae
l. laterale lineae asperae femoris
l. medialis lineae asperae femoris

la·brum *pl.* la·bra
l. acetabulare
l. articularis
glenoid l.
l. glenoidale
l. glenoidale articulationis coxae
l. glenoidale articulationis humeri

LAC
long-arm cast

lac·er·a·tion

la·cer·tus
l. fibrosus
l. fibrosus musculi bicipitis brachii
l. medius Weitbrechtii
l. medius Wrisbergii

La·cey
L. fully constrained device
L. Total Knee System

Lach·man
L. test

lac·tate de·hy·dro·gen·ase

la·cu·na *pl.* la·cu·nae
absorption l.
bone l.
cartilage l.
Howship l.
l. of muscles
l. musculorum
osseous l.
resorption l.

LAD
ligament augmentation device

La·gen·bach
L. elevator

Laing
L. concentric hip cup

LAI un·con·strained de·vice

Lam
L. modification of Jones procedure

Lam·bert
L.-Lowman bone clamp

Lam·bri·nu·di
L. procedure

la·mel·la *pl.* la·mel·lae
articular l.
basic l.
circumferential l.
concentric l.
endosteal l.
ground l.
haversian l.
intermediate l.
interstitial l.
osseous l.
periosteal l.
peripheral l.

lam·i·na *pl.* lam·i·nae
l. arcus vertebrae
bony l.
cribriform l.
cribriform l. of transverse fascia
l. fibrocartilaginea inter-pubica
interpubic l., fibrocartilag-inous
l. prevertebralis fasciae cervicalis

lam·i·na *(continued)*
   l. of vertebra
   l. of vertebral arch

lam·i·na·plas·ty

lam·i·nar

lam·i·nec·to·my
   bilateral l.
   decompression l.

lam·i·no·plas·ty

lam·i·not·o·my
   keyhole l.

La·my
   Maroteaux-L. mucopoly-
     saccharidosis syndrome
   Maroteaux-L. syndrome

Lan·dou·zy
   L. dystrophy
   L.-Dejerine disease

Land·smeer
   L. ligament

Lane
   L. bone holding forceps
   L's plate
   Murphy-L. bone skid

Lange
   Eden-L. procedure
   L. procedure
   L. reduction

Lan·gen·beck
   L's amputation
   L. periosteal elevator

Lan·gen·skiöld
   L. osteotomy
   L. procedure

Lan·ger
   L's axillary arch
   L. line
   L. mesomelic dysplasia
   L's muscle
   L.-Giedion syndrome

Lan·gor·ia
   L's sign

lap·a·rot·o·my

Lap·i·dus
   L. operation
   L. procedure

La·roc·ca
   Whitecloud and L. spinal
     fusion

Lar·rey
   L's amputation
   L's operation

Lar·sen
   L's syndrome
   Sinding-L.-Johansson dis-
     ease

La·sègue
   L. sign

la·ser

Lat·ar·jet
   Bristow-L. procedure

lat·er·al

la·tis·si·mus
   l. dorsi

la·tus *pl.* lat·e·ra
   metatarsus l.

Lauge
   L.-Hansen classification
     (for ankle fracture)

Lau·gier
   L's sign

Lau·rin
   L. angle
   L's projection

Lauth
   L's ligament

la·vage

law
> Meyer's l.
> Ollier's l.
> Teevan's l.
> Wolff's l.

lax·i·ty
> joint l.
> ligamentous l.

Lax·o·va
> Neu-L. syndrome

lay·er
> Dobie's l.
> fibrous l. of articular capsule
> Floegel's l.
> Ollier's l.
> osteogenetic l.
> synovial l. of articular capsule

LCP
> Legg-Calvé-Perthes disease

LCS To·tal Knee Sys·tem

LD
> lactate dehydrogenase

LE
> lupus erythematosus

lead
> serum l. level

Lead·bet·ter
> L. maneuver

LEAP
> Lewis expandable adjustable prosthesis

Le Den·tu
> L's suture

Leeds
> L. procedure

Le Fort
> L's amputation
> L. fracture

Le Fort (continued)
> L's suture

Leg
> leg amputation

leg
> badger l.
> baker l.
> bandy l.
> bayonet l.
> bow l.
> rider's l.
> scissor l.
> tennis l.

Legg
> L.-Calvé-Perthes disease

Leh·mann
> Börjeson-Forssman-L. syndrome

Leids
> L.-Keio ligament

Lein·bach
> L. screw

Lek·sell
> L. rongeur

LE (lupus erythematosus) prep

Lem·li
> Smith-L.-Opitz syndrome

length
> step l.
> stride l.
> wave l.

leng·then·ing
> Achilles tendon l.
> tendo Achillis l.
> thumb distraction l.
> Z-l.

length-sta·ble

length-un·sta·ble

Len·ox Hill brace

Len·ox Hill or·tho·sis

Lenz
    L.-Majewski hyperostosis
        syndrome
    L.-Majewski syndrome

L'Epis·cope Za·cha·ry
    L'E.Z. procedure

lep·to·dac·ty·lous

lep·to·dac·ty·ly

lep·to·me·nin·gi·tis

lep·to·men·in·gop·a·thy

Le·ri
    L's pleonosteosis
    L. sign
    L.-Weill dyschondrosteosis

Le·rich
    L's treatment

Le·riche
    L's disease

Le·roy
    L. I-cell syndrome

le·sion
    Bankart l.
    bone l.
    Galeazzi l.
    Galeazzi-equivalent l.
    Gaucher's l's
    Hill-Sachs l.
    impaction l.
    Monteggia l.
    Monteggia-equivalent l.
    onion scale l.
    onionskin l.
    SLAP (superior labrum
        anterior to posterior) l.
    soft tissue l.
    space-occupying l.
    uncommitted metaphyseal
        l.
    wire-loop l.

Let·ter·er
    L.-Siwe disease

le·va·tor *pl.* le·va·to·res
    l. scapulae

Le·vin
    Jarcho-L. syndrome

Le·vy
    L.-Hollister syndrome

Lew·in
    L. bone holding clamp

Lew·is
    L. expandable adjustable
        prosthesis
    L. nail
    L. and Chekofsky proce-
        dure
    Marcove, L., and Horos
        procedure

Lex·an jack·et

Ley·dig
    L's cylinders

Lher·mitte
    L's sign

Lib·er·a·tor
    L. elevator

Lich·ten·stern
    L. sign

li·do·caine

Lie·big
    Radley, L., and Brown ap-
        proach
    Radley, L., and Brown
        procedure

Lie·bolt
    L. procedure

lig·a·ment
    accessory l.
    accessory l's, plantar
    accessory l's, volar
    accessory l. of humerus
    accessory l's of metacarpo-
        phalangeal joints
    acromioclavicular l.

lig·a·ment *(continued)*

    acromiocoracoid l.

    adipose l. of knee (of Cruveilhier)

    alar l's

    alar l's of knee

    annular l., dorsal common

    annular l., inferior

    annular l., internal

    annular l. of ankle, external

    annular l. of ankle, internal

    annular l. of carpus, posterior

    annular l's of digits of foot

    annular l's of digits of hand

    annular l. of femur

    annular l's of fingers

    annular l. of malleolus, external

    annular l. of malleolus, internal

    annular l. of radius

    annular l. of tarsus, anterior

    annular l's of tendon sheaths of fingers

    annular l's of toes

    annular l. of wrist, dorsal posterior

    anterior cruciate l.

    anterior l. of head of fibula

    anterior l. of head of rib

    anterior longitudinal l.

    anterior sacroiliac l.

    anterior l. of neck of rib

    anterior l. of radiocarpal joint

    l. of antibrachium (of Weitbrecht)

    apical l's

    apical dental l.

    apical odontoid l.

    arcuate l's

    arcuate l., pubic

    arcuate l. of knee

lig·a·ment *(continued)*

    arcuate l. of pubis, inferior

    articular l. of vertebrae

    artificial l.

    atlantooccipital l., anterior

    atlantooccipital l., deep

    atlantooccipital l., lateral

    atlantooccipital l., posterior

    Barkow's l.

    Bellini's l.

    Bertin's l.

    Bichat's l.

    bifurcate l.

    bifurcate l's, deep

    bifurcate l's of Arnold, deep

    Bigelow's l.

    bigeminate l's of Arnold

    Bourgery's l.

    brachiocubital l.

    brachioradial l.

    Brodie's l.

    calcaneocuboid l.

    calcaneocuboid l., plantar

    calcaneofibular l.

    calcaneonavicular l.

    calcaneonavicular l., dorsal

    calcaneonavicular l., plantar

    calcaneotibial l.

    Caldani's l.

    Campbell's l.

    capitohamate l.

    capitotriquetral l.

    capitular l., volar

    capsular l's

    capsular l., internal

    carpal l.

    carpal l., dorsal

    carpal l., radiate

    carpometacarpal l's, anterior

    carpometacarpal l's, dorsal

    carpometacarpal l's, palmar

lig·a·ment *(continued)*

carpometacarpal l's, posterior

carpometacarpal l's, volar

cervical l., anterior

cervical l., posterior

cervical l. of sinus tarsi

cervicobasilar l.

check l's of axis

chondrosternal l., interarticular

chondroxiphoid l's

clavicular l., external capsular

Cleland's l.

coccygeal l., superior

collateral l.

collateral l., fibular

collateral l., radial

collateral l., radial carpal

collateral l., tibial

collateral l., ulnar

collateral l., ulnar carpal

collateral l. of carpus, radial

collateral l. of carpus, ulnar

collateral l's of interphalangeal articulations of foot

collateral l's of interphalangeal articulations of hand

collateral l's of metacarpophalangeal articulations

collateral l's of metatarsophalangeal articulations

Colles' l.

common l. of knee (of Weber)

common l. of wrist joint, deep

conoid l.

coracoacromial l.

coracoclavicular l.

coracoclavicular l., external

lig·a·ment *(continued)*

coracoclavicular l., internal

coracohumeral l.

coracoid l. of scapula

coronary l. of radius

costocentral l., anterior

costocentral l., interarticular

costoclavicular l.

costocoracoid l.

costosternal l's, radiate

costotransverse l.

costotransverse l., anterior

costotransverse l., lateral

costotransverse l., posterior

costotransverse l., superior

costotransverse l. of Krause, posterior

costovertebral l.

costoxiphoid l's

cotyloid l.

Cowper's l.

crucial l's of fingers

crucial l. of foot

cruciate l.

cruciate l. of atlas

cruciate l's of fingers

cruciate l's of knee

cruciate l. of knee, anterior

cruciate l. of knee, posterior

cruciate l. of leg

cruciate l's of toes

cruciform l. of atlas

crural l.

Cruveilhier's l's

cubitoradial l.

cubitoulnar l.

cuboideometatarsal l's, short

cuboideonavicular l., dorsal

cuboideonavicular l., oblique

lig·a·ment *(continued)*
    cuboideonavicular l., plantar
    cubonavicular l.
    cuboscaphoid l., plantar
    cuneocuboid l., dorsal
    cuneocuboid l., interosseous
    cuneocuboid l., plantar
    cuneometatarsal l's, interosseous
    cuneonavicular l's, dorsal
    cuneonavicular l's, plantar
    cutaneophalangeal l's
    cutaneous l. of fingers
    deep collateral l.
    deep transverse metacarpal l.
    deltoid l.
    deltoid l. of ankle
    deltoid l. of elbow
    Denucé's l.
    dorsal l's, carpal
    dorsal l., talonavicular
    dorsal l's of bases of metacarpal bones
    dorsal l's of bases of metatarsal bones
    dorsal l. of radiocarpal joint
    dorsal l's of tarsus
    dorsal l. of wrist
    external l's of Barkow, plantar
    fabellofibular l.
    falciform l.
    fallopian l.
    l. of Fallopius
    fibrous l., anterior
    fibrous l., posterior
    flaval l's
    Flood's l.
    Gerdy's l.
    glenohumeral l's
    glenoid l's of Cruveilhier
    glenoid l. of humerus
    glenoid l. of Macalister
    Grayson's l.

lig·a·ment *(continued)*
    hamatometacarpal l.
    l. of head of femoral bone
    l. of head of femur
    Henle's l.
    l's of Henry and Wrisberg
    Humphry's l.
    iliocostal l.
    iliofemoral l.
    iliolumbar l.
    iliopectineal l.
    iliopubic l.
    iliosacral l's, anterior
    iliosacral l's, interosseous
    iliosacral l., long
    iliotibial l. of Maissiat
    iliotrochanteric l.
    inferior l. of neck of rib of Henle
    inferior l. of tubercle of rib
    inferior glenohumeral l.
    inguinal l.
    inguinal l., external
    inguinal l., internal
    inguinal l., reflex
    interarticular l.
    interarticular l. of articulation of humerus
    interarticular l. of head of rib
    interarticular l. of hip joint
    interarticular sternocostal l.
    intercarpal l's, dorsal
    intercarpal l's, interosseous
    intercarpal l's, palmar
    intercarpal l's, volar
    interclavicular l.
    intercostal l's, external
    intercostal l's, internal
    intercuneiform l's, dorsal
    intercuneiform l's, interosseous
    intercuneiform l's, plantar
    intermetacarpal l's, anterior

lig·a·ment *(continued)*

intermetacarpal l's, distal
intermetacarpal l's, dorsal
intermetacarpal l's, interosseous
intermetacarpal l's, palmar
intermetacarpal l's, proximal, anterior
intermetacarpal l's, proximal, posterior
intermetacarpal l's, transverse, dorsal
intermetacarpal l's, transverse, volar
intermetatarsal l's, interosseous
intermetatarsal l's, plantar, distal
intermetatarsal l's, proximal, dorsal
intermetatarsal l's, proximal, plantar
intermetatarsal l's, transverse, dorsal
intermetatarsal l's, transverse, plantar
intermuscular l., fibular
intermuscular l. of arm, external
intermuscular l. of arm, internal
intermuscular l. of arm, lateral
intermuscular l. of arm, medial
intermuscular l. of thigh, external
intermuscular l. of thigh, lateral
intermuscular l. of thigh, medial
internal l. of neck of rib
interosseous l., radioulnar
interosseous l's, transverse metacarpal
interosseous l's of Barkow, internal

lig·a·ment *(continued)*

interosseous l's of bases of metacarpal bones
interosseous l's of bases of metatarsal bones
interosseous l. of Cruveilhier, costovertebral
interosseous l. of Cruveilhier, transversocostal
interosseous l's of knee
interosseous l. of leg
interosseous l. of pubis
interosseous l's of tarsus
l's of interphalangeal articulations of foot, plantar
l's of interphalangeal articulations of hand, palmar
interprocess l.
interpubic l.
interspinal l's
interspinous l's
intertarsal l's, dorsal
intertarsal l's, interosseous
intertarsal l's, plantar
intertransverse l's
intervertebral l.
intraarticular l. of head of rib
intrinsic l.
ischiocapsular l.
ischiofemoral l.
ischiosacral l's
laciniate l.
laciniate l., external
lambdoid l.
Landsmeer l.
lateral l. of ankle joint
lateral l. of carpus, radial
lateral l. of carpus, ulnar
lateral collateral l.
lateral l's of joints of fingers
lateral l's of joints of toes
lateral l. of knee
lateral meniscofemoral l.

lig·a·ment *(continued)*

   lateral l's of metacarpophalangeal joints

   lateral l's of metatarsophalangeal joints

   lateral l. of wrist joint, external

   lateral l. of wrist joint, internal

   Lauth's l.

   Leids-Keio l.

   Lisfranc's l.

   longitudinal l., anterior

   longitudinal l. of interspinal disk

   longitudinal l., posterior

   lumbocostal l.

   lunotriquetral l.

   l. of Maissiat

   Mauchart's l's

   l. of Mayer

   medial collateral l.

   medial l. of elbow joint

   medial l. of wrist

   meniscofemoral l., anterior

   meniscofemoral l., posterior

   metacarpal l's, dorsal

   metacarpal l's, interosseous

   metacarpal l's, palmar

   metacarpal l's, transverse,
deep

   metacarpal l., transverse,
superficial

   metacarpophalangeal l's,
anterior

   metacarpophalangeal l's,
palmar

   l's of metacarpophalangeal
articulations, palmar

   metatarsal l., anterior

   metatarsal l's, dorsal

   metatarsal l's, interosseus

   metatarsal l's, lateral

   metatarsal l's, lateral (of
Weitbrecht)

lig·a·ment *(continued)*

   metatarsal l's, lateral
proper (of Weber)

   metatarsal l's, plantar

   metatarsal l., transverse,
deep

   metatarsal l., transverse,
interosseous

   metatarsal l., transverse,
superficial

   metatarsophalangeal l's,
inferior

   l's of metatarsophalangeal
articulations, plantar

   middle glenohumeral l.

   middle l. of neck of rib

   mucous l.

   l. of nape

   navicularicuneiform l's,
plantar

   nuchal l.

   oblique l.

   oblique l. of Cooper

   oblique l. of forearm

   oblique l's of knee

   oblique l. of knee, posterior

   oblique l. of scapula

   oblique l. of superior radioulnar joint

   obturator l., atlantooccipi-
tal

   obturator l. of atlas

   occipitoaxial l.

   occipitoodontoid l's

   odontoid l., middle

   odontoid l's of axis

   orbicular l.

   orbicular l. of radius

   palmar l's

   palmar l., transverse, deep

   palmar l. of carpus

   palmar l. of radiocarpal
joint

   paravertebral l's

   patellar l.

   patellar l., internal

   patellar l., lateral

lig·a·ment *(continued)*
    pelvic l., posterior, great
    pelvic l., posterior, short
    pisimetacarpal l.
    pisohamate l.
    pisometacarpal l.
    pisounciform l.
    pisouncinate l.
    plantar l's
    plantar l., long
    plantar l. of second meta-
      tarsal bone
    plantar l. of tarsus
    popliteal l., arcuate
    popliteal l., external
    popliteal l., oblique
    posterior cruciate l.
    posterior l. of head of fib-
      ula
    posterior longitudinal l.
    posterior l. of radiocarpal
      joint
    Poupart's l.
    prismatic l. of Weitbrecht
    proper l's of costal carti-
      lages
    prosthetic l.
    proximal tibiofibular l.
    pubic l., inferior
    pubic l., superior
    pubic l. of Cowper
    pubic l. of Cruveilhier, an-
      terior
    pubocapsular l.
    pubofemoral l.
    quadrate l.
    radial l., lateral
    radial collateral l.
    radial l. of cubitocarpal ar-
      ticulation
    radiate l.
    radiate l., lateral
    radiate l. of carpus
    radiate l. of head of rib
    radiate l. of Mayer
    radiocapitate l.
    radiocarpal l., anterior
    radiocarpal l., dorsal

lig·a·ment *(continued)*
    radiocarpal l., palmar
    radiocarpal l., volar
    radioscaphocapitate l.
    radioscaphoid l.
    radiotriquetral l.
    reflex l. of Gimbernat
    reinforcing l's
    rhomboid l. of clavicle
    rhomboid l. of wrist
    ring l. of hip joint
    Robert's l.
    round l. of acetabulum
    round l. of Cloquet
    round l. of femur
    round l. of forearm
    rupture of l.
    sacciform l.
    sacrococcygeal l., anterior
    sacrococcygeal l., dorsal,
      deep
    sacrococcygeal l., dorsal,
      superficial
    sacrococcygeal l., lateral
    sacrococcygeal l., posterior,
      deep
    sacrococcygeal l., posterior,
      superficial
    sacrococcygeal l., ventral
    sacroiliac l's, anterior
    sacroiliac l's, dorsal
    sacroiliac l's, interosseous
    sacroiliac l's, posterior
    sacroiliac l's, ventral
    sacrosciatic l., anterior
    sacrosciatic l., great
    sacrosciatic l., internal
    sacrosciatic l., least
    sacrospinal l.
    sacrospinous l.
    sacrotuberal l.
    sacrotuberous l.
    scaphocuneiform l's, plan-
      tar
    scapholunate l.
    scaphotrapezial l.
    l. of Scarpa
    Schlemm's l's

lig·a·ment *(continued)*
   short lateral l.
   short plantar l.
   sphenoidal l., external
   sphenoideotarsal l's
   spinoglenoid l.
   spinosacral l.
   spring l.
   stellate l., anterior
   sternoclavicular l., anterior
   sternoclavicular l., posterior
   sternocostal l's
   sternocostal l., interarticular
   sternocostal l., intra-articular
   sternocostal l's, radiate
   l. of Struthers
   subflaval l.
   subpubic l.
   superficial l. of carpus
   superficial collateral l.
   superficial transverse intermetacarpal l.
   superior glenohumeral l.
   superior l. of hip
   superior l. of neck of rib, anterior
   superior l. of neck of rib, external
   suprascapular l.
   supraspinal l's
   supraspinous l's
   suspensory l., marsupial
   suspensory l. of axilla
   suspensory l. of axis
   suspensory l. of humerus
   synovial l.
   synovial l. of hip
   synthetic l.
   talocalcaneal l., interosseous
   talocalcaneal l., lateral
   talocalcaneal l., medial
   l. of talocrural joint, lateral

lig·a·ment *(continued)*
   talofibular l., anterior
   talofibular l., posterior
   talonavicular l.
   talotibial l., anterior
   talotibial l., posterior
   tarsal l., anterior
   tarsometatarsal l's, dorsal
   tarsometatarsal l's, plantar
   tendinotrochanteric l.
   tibiocalcaneal l.
   tibiocalcanean l.
   tibiofibular l.
   tibiofibular l., anterior
   tibiofibular l., posterior
   tibionavicular l.
   transverse l. of acetabulum
   transverse atlantal l.
   transverse l. of atlas
   transverse carpal l.
   transverse l. of carpus
   transverse humeral l.
   transverse l. of knee
   transverse l. of leg
   transverse l. of little head of rib
   transverse l. of scapula, inferior
   transverse l. of scapula, superior
   transverse l. of tibia
   transverse l. of wrist
   transverse l's of wrist, dorsal
   transversocostal l., superior
   trapezoid l.
   triangular l. of abdomen
   triangular l. of pubis, anterior
   triangular l. of scapula
   triangular l. of thigh
   trigeminate l's of Arnold
   triquetral l.
   triquetral l. of foot
   triquetral l. of scapula

lig·a·ment *(continued)*
    trochlear l.
    trochlear l's of foot
    trochlear l's of hand
    trochlear l's of little heads
      of metacarpal bones
    tuberososacral l.
    ulnar l. of carpus
    ulnar collateral l.
    ulnar l., lateral
    ulnocarpal l., palmar
    vaginal l's of fingers
    vaginal l's of toes
    l's of vaginal sheaths of
      fingers
    l's of vaginal sheaths of
      toes
    vertebropleural l.
    l. of Vesalius
    volar carpal l.
    volar l. of carpus, proper
    volar radiocarpal l.
    volar l. of wrist, anterior
    Walther's oblique l.
    web l.
    Weitbrecht's l.
    Winslow's l.
    Wrisberg's l.
    xiphicostal l's of Macalis-
      ter
    xiphoid l's
    Y l.
    yellow l's
    zonal l. of thigh

lig·a·men·tous

lig·a·men·tum *pl.* lig·a·men·
  ta
    l. acromioclaviculare
    ligamenta alaria
    ligamenta annularia digi-
      torum manus
    ligamenta annularia digi-
      torum pedis
    l. annulare radii
    l. apicis dentis axis
    l. apicis dentis epistrophei
    l. arcuatum pubis

lig·a·men·tum *(continued)*
    l. atlanto-occipitale anter-
      ius
    l. atlanto-occipitale later-
      ale
    l. bifurcatum
    l. calcaneocuboideum
    l. calcaneocuboideum plan-
      tare
    l. calcaneofibulare
    l. calcaneonaviculare
    l. calcaneonaviculare dor-
      sale
    l. calcaneonaviculare plan-
      tare
    l. calcaneotibiale
    l. capitis costae intra-ar-
      ticulare
    l. capitis costae radiatum
    l. capitis femoris
    l. capitis fibulae anterius
    l. capitis fibulae posterius
    l. capituli costae radiatum
    ligamenta capituli fibulae
    ligamenta capsularia
    l. carpi dorsale
    l. carpi radiatum
    l. carpi transversum
    l. carpi volare
    ligamenta carpometacar-
      palia dorsalia
    ligamenta carpometacar-
      palia palmaria
    ligamenta carpometacar-
      pea dorsalia
    ligamenta carpometacar-
      pea palmaria
    ligamenta collateralia ar-
      ticulationum digitorum
      manus
    ligamenta collateralia ar-
      ticulationum digitorum
      pedis
    ligamenta collateralia ar-
      ticulationum interphal-
      angealium manus
    ligamenta collateralia ar-
      ticulationum interphal-
      angealium pedis

lig·a·men·tum *(continued)*
  ligamenta collateralia ar-
    ticulationum metacarpo-
    phalangealium
  ligamenta collateralia ar-
    ticulationum metatarso-
    phalangealium
  l. collaterale carpi radiale
  l. collaterale carpi ulnare
  l. collaterale fibulare
  l. collaterale radiale
  l. collaterale tibiale
  l. collaterale ulnare
  l. colli costae
  l. conoideum
  l. coracoacromiale
  l. coracoclaviculare
  l. coracohumerale
  l. costoclaviculare
  l. costotransversarium
  l. costotransversarium lat-
    erale
  l. costotransversarium su-
    perius
  ligamenta costoxiphoidea
  l. cruciatum anterius genu
  l. cruciatum anterius ge-
    nus
  l. cruciatum atlantis
  l. cruciatum cruris
  ligamenta cruciata digito-
    rum manus
  ligamenta cruciata digito-
    rum pedis
  ligamenta cruciata genu
  ligamenta cruciata genus
  l. cruciatum posterius
    genu
  l. cruciatum posterius ge-
    nus
  l. cruciforme atlantis
  l. cuboideonaviculare dor-
    sale
  l. cuboideonaviculare plan-
    tare
  l. cuneocuboideum dorsale
  l. cuneocuboideum interos-
    seum

lig·a·men·tum *(continued)*
  l. cuneocuboideum plan-
    tare
  ligamenta cuneometatar-
    salia interossea
  ligamenta cuneometatar-
    sea interossea
  ligamenta cuneonavicu-
    laria dorsalia
  ligamenta cuneonavicu-
    laria plantaria
  l. deltoideum
  ligamenta extracapsularia
  ligamenta flava
  ligamenta glenohumeralia
  l. iliofemorale
  l. iliolumbale
  l. inguinale
  l. inguinale [Pouparti]
  l. inguinale reflexum
  l. inguinale reflexum [Col-
    lesi]
  ligamenta intercarpalia
    dorsalia
  ligamenta intercarpalia
    interossea
  ligamenta intercarpalia
    palmaria
  ligamenta intercarpea dor-
    salia
  ligamenta intercarpea in-
    terossea
  ligamenta intercarpea pal-
    maria
  l. interclaviculare
  ligamenta intercostalia
  ligamenta intercostalia ex-
    terna
  ligamenta intercostalia in-
    terna
  ligamenta intercuneifor-
    mia dorsalia
  ligamenta intercuneifor-
    mia interossea
  ligamenta intercuneifor-
    mia plantaria
  ligamenta interspinalia

lig·a·men·tum *(continued)*
    ligamenta intertransver-
      saria
    ligamenta intracapsularia
    l. ischiocapsulare
    l. ischiofemorale
    l. laciniatum
    l. laterale articulationis
      talocruralis
    l. longitudinale anterius
    l. longitudinale posterius
    l. lumbocostale
    l. malleoli lateralis anter-
      ius
    l. malleoli lateralis poster-
      ius
    l. mediale articulationis
      talocruralis
    l. meniscofemorale anter-
      ius
    l. meniscofemorale poster-
      ius
    ligamenta metacarpalia
      dorsalia
    ligamenta metacarpalia
      interossea
    ligamenta metacarpalia
      palmaria
    l. metacarpale transver-
      sum superficiale
    ligamenta metacarpea dor-
      salia
    ligamenta metacarpea in-
      terossea
    ligamenta metacarpea pal-
      maria
    l. metacarpeum transver-
      sum profundum
    l. metacarpeum transver-
      sum superficiale
    ligamenta metatarsalia
      dorsalia
    ligamenta metatarsalia in-
      terossea
    ligamenta metatarsalia
      plantaria
    l. metatarsale transver-
      sum profundum

lig·a·men·tum *(continued)*
    l. metatarsale transver-
      sum superficiale
    ligamenta metatarsea dor-
      salia
    ligamenta metatarsea in-
      terossea
    ligamenta metatarsea
      plantaria
    l. metatarseum transver-
      sum profundum
    l. metatarseum transver-
      sum superficiale
    l. mucosum
    ligamenta navicularicu-
      neiformia dorsalia
    ligamenta navicularicu-
      neiformia plantaria
    l. nuchae
    ligamenta palmaria arti-
      culationum interphalan-
      gealium manus
    ligamenta palmaria arti-
      culationum metacarpo-
      phalangealium
    l. patellae
    l. pisohamatum
    l. pisometacarpeum
    ligamenta plantaria arti-
      culationum interphalan-
      gealium pedis
    ligamenta plantaria arti-
      culationum metatarso-
      phalangealium
    l. plantare longum
    l. popliteum arcuatum
    l. popliteum obliquum
    l. pubicum superius
    l. pubocapsulare
    l. pubofemorale
    l. quadratum
    l. radiocarpale dorsale
    l. radiocarpale palmare
    l. radiocarpeum dorsale
    l. radiocarpeum palmare
    l. sacrococcygeum anterius
    l. sacrococcygeum dorsale
      profundum

lig·a·men·tum *(continued)*
   l. sacrococcygeum dorsale superficiale
   l. sacrococcygeum laterale
   l. sacrococcygeum posterius profundum
   l. sacrococcygeum posterius superficiale
   l. sacrococcygeum ventrale
   ligamenta sacroiliaca anteriora
   ligamenta sacroiliaca dorsalia
   ligamenta sacroiliaca interossea
   ligamenta sacroiliaca posteriora
   ligamenta sacroiliaca ventralia
   ligamenta sacrospinalia
   l. sacrospinosum
   l. sacrotuberale
   l. sacrotuberosum
   l. sternoclaviculare
   l. sternoclaviculare anterius
   l. sternoclaviculare posterius
   l. sternocostale interarticulare
   l. sternocostale intra-articulare
   ligamenta sternocostalia radiata
   l. supraspinale
   l. talocalcaneare interosseum
   l. talocalcaneare laterale
   l. talocalcaneare mediale
   l. talocalcaneum interosseum
   l. talocalcaneum laterale
   l. talocalcaneum mediale
   l. talofibulare anterius
   l. talofibulare posterius
   l. talonaviculare
   l. talonaviculare [dorsale]
   l. talotibiale anterius

lig·a·men·tum *(continued)*
   l. talotibiale posterius
   ligamenta tarsi dorsalia
   ligamenta tarsi interossea
   ligamenta tarsi plantaria
   ligamenta tarsometarsalia dorsalia
   ligamenta tarsometatarsalia plantaria
   ligamenta tarsometatarsea dorsalia
   ligamenta tarsometatarsea plantaria
   l. teres femoris
   l. tibiofibulare anterius
   l. tibiofibulare posterius
   l. tibionaviculare
   l. transversum acetabuli
   l. transversum atlantis
   l. transversum cruris
   l. transversum genus
   l. transversum scapulae inferius
   l. transversum scapulae superius
   l. trapezoideum
   l. tuberculi costae
   l. ulnocarpale palmare
   l. ulnocarpeum palmare
   ligamenta vaginalia digitorum manus
   ligamenta vaginalia digitorum pedis

li·ga·tion

lig·a·ture

limb
   congenital l. absence
   lower l.
   l. salvage
   terminal transverse l. absence
   upper l.

limb-spar·ing

lim·bus *pl.* lim·bi
   l. acetabuli

lim·bus *(continued)*
   l. annularis

lim·it
   endurance l.
   fatigue l.

li·mo·ther·a·py

limp
   Trendelenburg l.

Lin·berg
   Tikhor-L. procedure

Lin·de·man
   L. procedure

Lin·der
   L. sign

Lind·holm
   L. procedure

line
   l. of Amici
   anterior humeral l.
   anterior spinal l.
   arcuate l. of ilium
   arcuate l. of pelvis
   basilar l. of Wackenheim
   Blumensaat l.
   Brücke's l's
   Bryant's l.
   cement l.
   Chamberlain's l.
   costoarticular l.
   curved l. of ilium
   curved l. of ilium, inferior
   curved l. of ilium, middle
   curved l. of ilium, superior
   Dobie's l.
   Duhot's l.
   epiphyseal l.
   Feiss' l.
   fracture l.
   Fränkel l.
   gluteal l.
   gluteal l., anterior
   gluteal l., inferior
   gluteal l., posterior
   growth arrest l.

line *(continued)*
   Harris l's
   Hensen's l.
   Heuter l.
   Holden's l.
   Hueter's l.
   iliopectineal l.
   intercondylar l.
   intercondyloid l.
   intertrochanteric l.
   intertrochanteric l., anterior
   intertrochanteric l., posterior
   Kilian's l.
   Köler's l.
   Krause's l.
   Langer's l's
   lead l.
   McGregor's l.
   McRae's l.
   Meyer's l.
   midspinal l.
   midsternal l.
   muscular l's of scapula
   Nélaton's l.
   oblique l. of femur
   oblique l. of fibula
   oblique l. of tibia
   Ogston's l.
   pectineal l.
   popliteal l. of femur
   popliteal l. of tibia
   posterior spinal l.
   quadrate l.
   radiocapitellar l.
   radiolucent l.
   rough l. of femur
   Shenton's l.
   soleal l. of tibia
   spinolaminar l. of Swischuk
   spiral l. of femur
   subscapular l's
   supracondylar l. of femur, lateral
   supracondylar l. of femur, medial

line *(continued)*
 l. supracondylaris lateralis femoris
 l. supracondylaris medialis femoris
 terminal l. of pelvis
 transischial l.
 transverse l. of sacral bone
 transverse l. of sacrum
 trapezoid l.
 Ullmann's l.
 Wackenheim's l.
 Wagner's l.
 white l. of pelvic fascia
 Wimberger's l.
 Wrisberg's l's
 Y-l.
 Z l.

lin·ea *pl.* lin·eae
 l. alba
 l. arcuata ossis ilii
 l. aspera
 l. aspera femoris
 l. epiphysialis
 l. glutea anterior
 l. glutea inferior
 l. glutea posterior
 l. iliopectinea
 l. innominata
 l. intercondylaris femoris
 l. intercondyloidea femoris
 l. intertrochanterica
 l. intertrochanterica posterior
 lineae musculares scapulae
 l. musculi solei
 l. obliqua fibulae
 l. obliqua tibiae
 l. pectinea femoris
 l. poplitea tibiae
 l. spiralis
 l. terminalis pelvis
 lineae transversae ossis sacri
 l. trapezoidea

lin·e·ar

lin·er
 bone l.

Ling
 L. total hip replacement

li·nin

lin·ing
 synovial l.

link·age
 four-bar l.
 track-bound l.

Link V pros·the·sis

Lin-Trol

lip
 acetabular l.
 articular l.
 external l. of iliac crest
 external l. of linea aspera of femur
 fibrocartilaginous l. of acetabulum
 glenoid l.
 glenoid l. of articulation of hip
 glenoid l. of articulation of humerus
 internal l. of iliac crest
 lateral l. of linea aspera of femur
 medial l. of linea aspera of femur
 posterior l. of acetabulum

lip·id

lipo·ar·thri·tis

lipo·fi·bro·ma

lipo·hem·ar·thro·sis

li·po·ma
 l. arborescens
 intraosseous l.
 spinal l.

lipo·sar·co·ma
 myxoid l.

lip·ping

Lipp·man
Cobb-L. technique

Lis·franc
L's amputation
L's dislocation
L. fracture
L's joint
L's ligament
L's operation
L's tubercle

Lis·ter
L's tubercle

Lis·ton
L's knife
L's splint
Stille-L. bone cutting for-
ceps

Lit·ler
Snow-L. procedure

lit·ter
Neal-Robertson l.

Lit·tle Lea·guer's el·bow

Lit·tle Lea·guer's shoul·der

Litt·ler
Eaton-L. arthroplasty
L. opponensplasty
L. pollicization

Lit·tle·wood
L. amputation

Liv·er·pool el·bow pros·the·
sis

Liv·er·pool un·con·strained
de·vice

LLC
long-leg cast

Lloyd-Rob·erts
L.-R. osteotomy
L.-R. procedure

LLWC
long-leg walking cast

load
compressive l.
dynamic l.
functional l.
ultimate l.

load·ing
axial l.

Lob·stein
L's disease
L's syndrome

Lo·cal·io
L. procedure

lo·cal·iz·er
Risser l.

lo·ca·tion
surface l.

lock
bail knee l.
dial l.
lateral spring-loaded l.

lock·ing

loc·u·lat·ed

Lo·dine

loge
l. de Guyon

log roll

Lon·don
L. elbow prosthesis

lon·gi·tu·di·nal

loop
perineal l.

Loose
L. procedure

loo·sen·ing
cup l.

Lo·pres·ti
Essex-L. fracture

Lo·pres·ti *(continued)*
    Essex-L. procedure

Lord
    L. total hip replacement

lor·do·sco·li·o·sis

lor·do·sis
    lumbar l.

lor·dot·ic

Lor·enz
    L's operation
    L's osteotomy
    L. reduction
    L. sign

Lor·en·zo
    L. screw

Lor·raine Day
    method of L.D.

Lo·see
    L. procedure

loss
    bone l.

Lot·ke
    Ecker, L., and Glazer tendon transfer

Lot·tes
    L. nail
    L. pin

Lou Geh·rig
    L.G's disease

loupe

Lowe
    L. syndrome
    L.-Miller elbow prosthesis

Low·man
    L. bone clamp
    L. bone clamp, modified
    L. procedure
    L. shelf procedure
    Lambert-L. bone clamp

Lowry
    Coffin-L. syndrome

lox·ar·thron

lox·ar·thro·sis

lox·ia

lox·ot·o·my

Lu·bi·nus
    L. arthroplasty
    L. hip
    L. SP II hip prosthesis
    L. unconstrained device

Lu·cas
    Abbott-Fisher-L. arthrodesis
    L. and Cottrell osteotomy
    L. and Murray arthrodesis

Lu·cite

Luck
    L. procedure
    L.-Bishop bone saw

Lud·loff
    L's sign
    L. procedure

Lu·er
    Stille-L. rongeur

Luft
    L's disease

lum·ba·go
    ischemic l.

lum·bar

lum·bar·iza·tion

lum·bo·dyn·ia

lum·bri·cal

lu·men *pl.* lu·mi·na

lu·na·re

lu·nate

lu·na·to·ma·la·cia

Lunce·ford
    L. total hip replacement

Lund
    L. unicompartmental de-
        vice

lu·no·tri·que·tral

lu·nu·la *pl.* lu·nu·lae
    l. of scapula

lu·pus
    discoid l.
    drug-induced l.
    l. erythematosus (LE)
    l. erythematosus, cuta-
        neous
    l. erythematosus, discoid
        (DLE)
    l. erythematosus, hyper-
        trophic
    l. erythematosus, systemic
        (SLE)
    l. erythematosus profun-
        dus
    l. erythematosus tumidus
    neonatal l.
    l. profundus
    systemic l. erythematosus
    transient neonatal sys-
        temic l. erythematosus

Luque
    Harri-L. technique
    L. instrumentation
    L.-Galveston instrumenta-
        tion

lurch
    abductor l.
    Trendelenburg l.

Lusch·ka
    L's joint
    joints of L.
    ligaments of L.

lux·a·tio
    l. coxae congenita
    l. erecta
    l. imperfecta
    l. perinealis

lux·a·tion
    Malgaigne's l.

Ly·man
    L.-Smith traction

Lyme bor·re·li·o·sis

Lyme dis·ease

lymph

lym·phan·gi·og·ra·phy

lym·pho·ma
    malignant l.
    osseous l.
    primary l.

Lyn·holm
    L. knee-scoring scale

Lynn
    L. procedure

Ly·ser
    trapezium bone of L.
    trapezoid bone of L.

Lys·holm
    L. knee score

ly·sis
    bone l.

lyt·ic

M
 muscle
M/3
 middle third
m.
 L. musculus (muscle)
Ma
 M. and Griffith procedure
Mc·Bride
 M. hip prosthesis
 M. procedure
Mc·Car·roll
 M. osteotomy
Mac·Car·thy
 M. procedure
Mc·Car·ty
 M. procedure
Mc·Cash
 M. procedure
Mc·Cau·ley
 M. procedure
Mc·Cune
 Albright-M.-Sternberg
  syndrome
 M.-Albright syndrome
Mc·Cut·chen
 Hydroxylapatite M. Total
  Hip System
 M. SLT Total Hip System
Mac·dow·el
 M's frenum
Mc·El·ven·ny
 M. procedure
mac·er·a·tion
Mac·ew·en
 M. and Shands osteotomy

Mc·Fad·din
 Spittler and M. amputa-
  tion
Mc·Far·land
 M. approach
Mc·Gre·gor
 M's line
Mc·Guire
 M. pelvic positioner
ma·chine
 continuous passive
  motion m.
Mac·In·tosh
 M. procedure
 M. test
 M. unicompartmental de-
  vice
Mc·Kee
 M. elbow prosthesis
 M.-Farrar total hip re-
  placement
Mc·Kee·ver
 M. procedure
 M. prosthesis
 Wilson and M. procedure
Mc·Ken·zie
 M. exercises
 M. extension exercises
Mac·ken·zie
 M's amputation
Mc·Ku·sick
 metaphyseal chondrodys-
  plasia, M. type
Mc·Laugh·lin
 M. plate
 M. procedure
 M. screw

Mc·Leod
  Boyd and M. procedure

Mac·Leod
  M's capsular rheumatism

Mc·Mas·ter
  M. graft

Mc·Mur·ray
  M. circumduction maneu-
    ver
  M. osteotomy
  M. sign

Mc·Nab
  M. criteria
  M's hidden zone

Mc·Rae
  M's line

Mc·Rey·nolds
  M. driver-extractor
  M. procedure

mac·ro·bra·chia

mac·ro·chei·ria

mac·ro·chi·ria

mac·ro·dac·tyl·ia

mac·ro·dac·ty·ly

mac·ro·po·dia

Mad·e·lung
  M's deformity
  M's disease

Mad·re·por·ic
  M. total hip replacement
  M. hip prosthesis

Maf·fuc·ci
  M. syndrome

Mag·an

ma·gen·ta
  m. O

mag·ne·si·um
  choline and m. salicylates
  m. salicylate

mag·ni·fi·ca·tion
  loupe m.

Mag·nu·son
  M. procedure
  M.-Stack procedure

main
  m. en crochet
  m. en griffe
  m. en lorgnette
  m. en singe
  m. en squelette

Mai·son·neuve
  M's amputation
  M. fracture
  M's sign

Mais·siat
  M's band
  iliotibial ligament of M.
  ligament of M.
  M's tract

Ma·jes·tro
  M., Ruda, and Frost proce-
    dure

Ma·jew·ski
  Lenz-M. hyperostosis syn-
    drome
  Lenz-M. syndrome
  short rib–polydactyly, M.
    type
  short rib–polydactyly, non-
    M. type
  metaplastic m.
  myeloplastic m.

mal·a·co·pla·kia

mal·a·co·sar·co·sis

mal·a·cos·te·on

mal·aise

mal·align·ment
  rotational m.

mal·ar·tic·u·la·tion

Ma·law·er
   M. procedure

mal·for·ma·tion
   arteriovenous m. (AVM)

Mal·gaigne
   M's amputation
   M. fracture
   M's luxation

ma·lig·nan·cy
   musculoskeletal m.
   small round-cell m's of
     bone

ma·lig·nant

Mal·is
   M. bipolar coagulator

mal·le·o·lar

mal·le·o·lus *pl.* mal·le·o·li
   external m.
   m. externus
   m. fibulae
   fibular m.
   inner m.
   internal m.
   m. internus
   lateral m.
   lateral m. of fibula
   m. lateralis
   m. lateralis fibulae
   medial m.
   medial m. of tibia
   m. medialis
   m. medialis tibiae
   outer m.
   posterior m.
   radial m.
   m. radialis
   m. tibiae
   tibial m.
   ulnar m.
   m. ulnaris

mal·le·ot·o·my

mal·let

Mal·lo·ry
   M.-Head Hip
   M.-Head prosthesis

mal·track·ing
   m. articulorum senilis
   m. senile
   m. vertebrale suboccipitale

mal·un·ion

Man·dol

ma·neu·ver
   Adson's m.
   Allen m.
   Allis m.
   Bigelow reverse m.
   circumduction m.
   Faber m.
   Fowler m.
   Jendrassik's m.
   Leadbetter m.
   McMurray's circumduc-
     tion m.
   Meyn and Quigley m.
   Parvin m.
   Patrick m.
   Phalen's m.
   reverse Bigelow m.
   Schreiber's m.
   Stimson m.
   Valsalva's m.

man·i·pha·lanx

ma·nip·u·la·tion
   joint m.

Man·ning
   Gill, M., and White lum-
     bar spinal fusion

ma·nu·bri·um *pl.* ma·nu·bria
   m. sterni
   m. of sternum

ma·nus *pl.* ma·nus
   m. cava
   m. extensa
   m. flexa
   m. plana

ma·nus *(continued)*
    m. superextensa
    m. valga
    m. vara

Ma·quet
    M. osteotomy
    M. procedure

Mar·che·sa·ni
    Weill-M. syndrome

Mar·cove
    M., Lewis, and Horos pro-
      cedure

Mar·cus
    M. classification (for avas-
      cular necrosis of femoral
      head)
    M., Balourdas, Heiple ar-
      throdesis

Mar·fan
    M's syndrome

mar·gin
    m. of acetabulum
    axillary m. of scapula
    cartilaginous m. of acetab-
      ulum
    discovertebral m.
    falciform m. of white line
      of pelvic fascia
    m. of fibula, anterior
    m. of fibula, posterior
    m. of foot, fibular
    m. of foot, lateral
    m. of foot, medial
    m. of humerus, lateral
    m. of humerus, medial
    infiltrative m.
    interosseous m. of fibula
    interosseous m. of tibia
    radial m. of forearm
    m. of radius, dorsal
    m. of scapula, anterior
    m. of scapula, external
    m. of scapula, lateral
    m. of scapula, superior
    m. of tibia, anterior

mar·gin *(continued)*
    m. of tibia, medial
    tibial m. of foot
    m. of ulna, anterior
    m. of ulna, dorsal
    m. of ulna, posterior
    ulnar m. of forearm
    vertebral m. of scapula
    volar m. of radius
    volar m. of ulna

mar·go *pl.* mar·gi·nes
    m. acetabuli
    m. anterior fibulae
    m. anterior radii
    m. anterior tibiae
    m. anterior ulnae
    m. axillaris scapulae
    m. dorsalis radii
    m. dorsalis ulnae
    m. fibularis pedis
    m. infraglenoidalis tibiae
    m. interosseus fibulae
    m. interosseus radii
    m. interosseus tibiae
    m. interosseus ulnae
    m. lateralis antebrachii
    margines laterales digito-
      rum pedis
    m. lateralis humeri
    m. lateralis pedis
    m. lateralis scapulae
    m. medialis antebrachii
    margines mediales digito-
      rum pedis
    m. medialis humeri
    m. medialis pedis
    m. medialis scapulae
    m. medialis tibiae
    m. pedis lateralis
    m. pedis medialis
    m. posterior fibulae
    m. posterior radii
    m. posterior ulnae
    m. radialis antebrachii
    m. radialis humeri
    m. superior scapulae
    m. tibialis pedis

mar·go *(continued)*
 m. ulnaris antebrachii
 m. ulnaris humeri
 m. vertebralis scapulae
 m. volaris radii
 m. volaris ulnae

Ma·rie
 Charcot-M.-Tooth disease
 M's disease
 M's hypertrophy
 M. syndrome
 M.-Bamberger disease
 M.-Charcot-Tooth disease
 M.-Foix sign
 M.-Strümpell disease
 M.-Strümpell spondylitis
 M.-Tooth disease
 Strümpell-M. disease

Mar·in·es·co
 M.-Sjögren syndrome

mark
 tide m.

mark·er
 femoral head m.
 suture m.

Mark·ham
 M.-Meyerding retractor

Mar·mor
 M. unconstrained device

Ma·ro·teaux
 M.-Lamy mucopolysaccha-
  ridosis syndrome
 M.-Lamy syndrome

mar·row
 bone m.
 bone m., red
 bone m., yellow
 bone m. biopsy
 bone m. transplant
 fat m.
 gelatinous m.
 red m.
 yellow m.

Mar·shall
 M. knee-grading scale
 M. procedure
 M. syndrome

mar·su·pi·al·iza·tion

mar·sup·i·um *pl.* mar·su·pia
 marsupia patellaris

Mar·tin
 M. bandage
 M's disease
 M. osteotomy
 M. procedure
 M. screw
 M. vigorimeter

Ma·son
 Koch-M. dressing
 M's classification (for ra-
  dial head fractures)

mass
 bone m.
 center of m.
 lateral m. of atlas
 lateral m. of cervical spine
 lateral m. of sacrum
 lateral m. of vertebrae
 presacral m.
 soft tissue m.

mas·sa *pl.* mas·sae
 m. lateralis atlantis
 m. lateralis ossis sacri
 m. lateralis vertebrae

Mas·sie
 M. driver
 M. extractor
 M. inserter
 M. nail

Mas·son
 M. stain

MAST
 military (medical) anti-
  shock trousers

mat
 differential pressure m.

mat *(continued)*
    Harris m.
    Harrison-Beath differential pressure m.

Match·ett
    M.-Brown hip prosthesis
    M.-Brown total hip replacement

ma·te·ri·al
    anisotropic m.

ma·tri·cec·to·my
    Steindler m.

ma·trix *pl.* ma·tri·ces
    bone m.
    germinal m.
    sarcoplasmic m.

Mat·ti
    M.-Russe graft

mat·u·ra·tion
    fusion m.

ma·tur·i·ty
    skeletal m.

Mauch
    Henschke-M. prosthesis

Mau·chart
    M's ligaments

Mauck
    M. procedure
    reverse M. procedure

Max·on
    M. suture

May·er
    ligament of M.
    radiate ligament of M.

May·field
    M. pin-holder headrest

Ma·yo
    M. ankle prosthesis
    M. clamp
    M. hip prosthesis
    M. hip score

Ma·yo *(continued)*
    M. procedure
    M. scissors
    M. total ankle replacement
    M.-Collins retractor
    M.-Thomas collar

Ma·yo Clin·ic hip rat·ing scale

Ma·zas
    M. elbow prosthesis

Ma·zur
    M. ankle rating

MC
    metacarpal amputation

MCH
    mean corpuscular hemoglobin

MCHC
    mean corpuscular hemoglobin concentration

MCL
    medial collateral ligament

MCV
    mean corpuscular volume

MD-50

MD-60

MD-76

mech·a·nism
    extensor m.
    quadriceps m.

Meck·el
    anterior tubercle of humerus of M.
    M.-Gruber syndrome

Me·clo·fen

me·clo·fen·am·ate

Me·clo·men

Meda Cap

Meda Tab

me·di·al

me·di·a·lis

me·di·al·iza·tion

med·i·cine
    physical and rehabilita-
      tion m.
    sports m.

me·dio·car·pal

me·dio·tar·sal

Med·i·pren

me·di·sca·le·nus

me·di·um *pl.* me·dia, me·di·
ums
    contrast m.

me·dul·la *pl.* me·dul·lae
    m. of bone
    m. ossium
    m. ossium flava
    m. ossium rubra

med·ul·li·tis

med·ul·li·za·tion

me·dul·lo·ar·thri·tis

Me·fox·in

Mega·cil·lin

meg·a·lo·chei·ria

meg·a·lo·dac·tyl·ia

meg·a·lo·dac·ty·lism

meg·a·lo·dac·ty·lous

meg·a·lo·dac·ty·ly

meg·a·lo·po·dia

mel·ag·ra

mel·al·gia

Mel·a·nie
    M. infection

Mel·chi·or
    Dyggve-M.-Clausen syn-
      drome

me·lis·so·ther·a·py

Mel·nick
    M.-Needles syndrome

melo·rhe·os·to·sis

melo·sal·gia

mem·bra

mem·bra·na *pl.* mem·bra·nae
    m. atlanto-occipitalis ante-
      rior
    m. atlanto-occipitalis pos-
      terior
    m. capsularis
    m. fibrosa capsulae articu-
      laris
    m. intercostalis externa
    m. intercostalis interna
    m. interossea antebrachii
    m. interossea cruris
    m. sacciformis
    m. sterni
    m. suprapleuralis
    m. synovialis capsulae ar-
      ticularis
    m. tectoria

mem·brane
    aponeurotic m.
    atlanto-occipital m., ante-
      rior
    atlanto-occipital m., poste-
      rior
    capsular m.
    costocoracoid m.
    cribriform m.
    fibrous m. of articular cap-
      sule
    ground m.
    intercostal m., external
    intercostal m., internal
    interosseous m.
    interosseous m. of forearm

mem·brane *(continued)*
  interosseous m., radioul-
    nar
  interosseous m. of leg
  interspinal m's
  Krause's m.
  ligamentous m.
  medullary m.
  oblique m. of forearm
  obturator m. of atlas, an-
    terior
  obturator m. of atlas, pos-
    terior
  occipitoaxial m., long
  sternal m.
  m. of sternum
  suprapleural m.
  synovial m.
  tectorial m.
  tendinous m.

Men·del
  M.-Bekhterev reflex

Men·est

me·nin·ges

me·nin·gi·o·ma

me·nin·gism

men·in·gis·mus

men·in·gi·tis *pl.* men·in·git·
  i·des

me·nin·go·cele

me·nin·go·en·ceph·a·lo·my·
  eli·tis

me·nin·go·my·eli·tis

me·nin·go-os·teo·phle·bi·tis

me·nin·go·sis

men·is·cec·to·my
  arthroscopic m.
  partial m.

men·is·ci·tis

me·nis·co·syn·o·vi·al

me·nis·cus *pl.* me·nis·ci
  m. of acromioclavicular
    joint
  articular m.
  m. articularis
  discoid m.
  discoid lateral m.
  m. of inferior radioulnar
    joint
  joint m.
  lateral m.
  lateral m. of knee joint
  m. lateralis articulationis
    genus
  medial m.
  medial m. of knee joint
  m. medialis articulationis
    genus
  regenerated medial m.
  m. of sternoclavicular joint
  tears of m.

Men·kes
  M. syndrome

Men·nell
  M. sign

Men·son
  M. and Scheck procedure

me·ral·gia

mer·cap·to·pu·rine

Mer·chant
  M. angle
  M's projection
  M. view

mero·myo·sin

mer·os·tot·ic

Mer·si·lene
  M. tape

meso·car·pal

meso·chon·dri·um

meso·cu·nei·form

meso·glu·te·al

meso·glu·te·us

meso·phrag·ma

meso·scap·u·la

meso·ster·num

meso·tar·sal

meso·the·nar

Mes·sen·baugh
Amspacher and M. osteot-
omy

meta-ar·thrit·ic

meta·car·pal

meta·car·pec·to·my

meta·car·po·pha·lan·ge·al

meta·car·pus

meta·phys·e·al

me·taph·y·ses

meta·phys·i·al

me·taph·y·sis *pl.* me·taph·y·
ses

meta·phys·itis

meta·pla·sia
chondroid m.
osseous m.

meta·plas·tic

meta·po·di·a·lia

met·apoph·y·sis

me·tas·ta·sis
calcareous m.
skip m.

me·tas·ta·size

meta·stat·ic

meta·ster·num

meta·tar·sal
dorsiflexed m.
plantarflexed m.

meta·tar·sal·gia

meta·tar·sec·to·my

meta·tar·so·pha·lan·ge·al

meta·tar·sus
m. adductocavus
m. adductovarus
m. adductus
m. atavicus
m. brevis
m. latus
m. primus varus
m. varus

meta·zo·nal

meth·ac·ry·late

meth·a·cy·cline

meth·a·nol

meth·od
Abbott's m.
Baer's m.
Charnley and DeLee m.
closed-plaster m.
Cloward m.
Cobb m.
Elmslie-Trillat m.
Fergusson m.
m. of Lorraine Day
modified Westergren m.
Orr m.
Ranawat's m.
Raney m.
Redlund-Johnell m.
rod-sleeve m.
Stullberg m.
trapdoor m.
Trueta m.

meth·o·trex·ate

meth·yl·meth·ac·ry·late

Me·ti·zol

Met·ric 21

me·triz·a·mide

Met·ro I.V.

me·tro·ni·da·zole

Met·zen·baum
    M. scissors

Meu·li
    M. arthroplasty
    M. wrist prosthesis

Mex·ate

Mey·er
    M's law
    M's line

Mey·er·ding
    Markham-M. retractor
    M. chisel
    M. gouge
    M. osteotome
    M's retractor

Meyn
    M. and Quigley maneuver

Mey·net
    M's nodes

Mez·lin

mez·lo·cil·lin

M/3 fracture

MG (Miller/Galante) Knee
    Sys·tem

MHP (Mallory-Head
    prosthesis) ac·e·tab·u·lar
    com·po·nent

Mi·chael Reese
    M.R. prosthesis
    M.R. Total Shoulder

Mi·che·le
    M. punch

mi·cro·ab·scess

mi·cro·dac·tyl·ia

mi·cro·dac·ty·ly

mi·cro·dis·kec·to·my
    arthroscopic m.
    posterolateral m.

mi·cro·frac·ture

mi·cro·in·stru·ment

mi·cro·in·ter·lock

mi·cro·lam·i·nec·to·my
    lateral m.
    posterior m.

mi·cro·mo·tion

mi·cros·ce·lous

mi·cros·co·py
    electron m.
    scanning electron m.
    transmission electron m.

mi·cro·sphere

mi·cro·sur·gery

mi·cro·vas·cu·lar

Mi·das Rex bur

mid·car·pal

middle/3

mid·foot

Mi·dol

mid·stance
    terminal s.

mid·ster·num

mid·tar·sal

Mie·tens
    M. syndrome

Mi·gnon
    M's eosinophilic granu-
        loma

mi·gra·tion
    foraminal m.
    prosthetic m.
    superior m.

Mik·u·licz
    M's angle
    M's operation
    Vladimiroff-M. amputation

Milch
    Darrach-Hughston-M.
        fracture
    M. procedure

Miles
    Dall-M. trochanteric clamp

Mil·gram
    M. test

Milk·man
    M's syndrome

Mil·lard
    Gillies and M. technique

Mil·ler
    Lowe-M. elbow prosthesis
    M's disease
    M. procedure
    M. syndrome
    M.-Dieker syndrome
    M.-Galante (MG) Knee
        System
    Phalen-M. opponensplasty

Mills
    M. test

Mil·roy
    M's disease

Mil·wau·kee cer·vi·co·tho·
    ra·co·lum·bo·sa·cral or·
    tho·sis

Mil·wau·kee or·tho·sis

Mil·wau·kee shoul·der

Mil·wau·kee TLSO

Min·er·va
    M. jacket
    M. plaster

mini·ar·throt·o·my

Min·ne·so·ta Rate of Ma·nip·
    u·la·tion Test

Minns
    M. knee prosthesis

mi·no·cau·sal·gia

Mi·no·cin

mi·no·cy·cline

Mi·nor
    M. sign
    M. procedure

mir·ror hand

MIS
    minimal intervention sur-
        gery

mi·so·pros·tol

Mitch·ell
    M. operation

mi·tel·la

Mit·tel·mei·er
    M. hip prosthesis

Mi·ya·ka·wa
    M. procedure
    M. technique

Mo·berg
    M. arthrodesis

Mo·bi·din

mo·bil·i·ty
    functional m.

mo·bi·li·za·tion
    joint m.

mod·u·lar

mod·u·lar·i·ty

mod·i·fi·ca·tion
    Lam m. of Jones procedure
    shoe m.

mod·u·lus
    elastic m.
    m. of elasticity
    shear m.

Moe
    Bickel and M. tendon
        transfer
    M. intertrochanteric plate
    M. plate

Moe *(continued)*
    M. sacral hooks

mogi·ar·thria

Mohr
    M. syndrome

mold
    Aufranc concentric hip m.

mole·skin

mol·le
    heloma m.

mol·li·ti·es
    m. ossium

mo·lyb·den·um

mo·ment
    bending m.
    flexion m.
    m. of inertia
    mass m. of inertia
    Poland m. of inertia

mo·men·tum

mon·ar·thric

mon·ar·thri·tis
    m. deformans

mon·ar·tic·u·lar

Möncke·berg
    M's sclerosis

Mo·nel

Monk
    M. total hip replacement

mono·ar·thri·tis

mono·ar·tic·u·lar

Mon·o·cid

mono·fil·a·ment
    Simms-Weinstein m.

Mono-Ge·sic

mono·mel·ic

mono·myo·si·tis

mono-os·te·it·ic

mono·so·di·um urate

mon·os·tot·ic

Mon·ro
    M's bursa

Mon·teg·gia
    M's dislocation
    M.-equivalent lesion
    M's fracture
    M. fracture-dislocation
    M. lesion

Mon·ter·caux
    M. fracture

Mon·ti·cel·li
    M.-Spinelli fixation device

Moore
    Austin-M. hip prosthesis
    B.H.M. procedure
    J.R.M. procedure
    M's fracture
    M. hip prosthesis
    M. osteotomy
    M. pin
    M. plate
    M. procedure
    M. prosthesis extractor

mor·bid·i·ty

mor·bus
    m. coxae senilis

mor·cel·lat·ed

mor·cel·la·tion

Mo·rel
    M. syndrome
    Stewart-M. syndrome

Mor·es·tin
    M. amputation

Mo·ro
    M. reflex
    Ruiz-M. procedure

Mor·quio
    M. sign
    M's syndrome

Mor·scher
    M. hip prosthesis

Mor·ton
    M. foot
    M. neuroma
    M's syndrome
    M. test

MOSC (Miami Orthopaedic Surgical Clinics) pros·the·sis

Mose
    M. concentric ring

moth-eat·en

mo·tion
    continuous passive m. (CPM)
    helical axis of m.
    joint m.
    range of m.
    plastic m.

Mo·trin

mound·ing

mouse
    joint m.

mouth
    tapir m.

move·ment
    gliding m.
    hinge m.

mov·er
    prime m.

mox·a·lac·tam

Mox·am

Mo·zer
    M's disease

MP
    metacarpophalangeal

MP *(continued)*
    metaphalangeal
    metatarsophalangeal

MPI

MPI MDP

MPI Py·ro·phos·phate

MP35N

MP stop

MRI
    magnetic resonance imaging

MRTS
    Michael Reese Total Shoulder

MSBOS
    maximal surgical blood order schedule

MT
    metatarsal
    metatarsal amputation

mu·co·poly·sac·cha·ride

mu·co·poly·sac·cha·ri·do·sis

mu·co·pu·ru·lent

mu·co·san·guin·e·ous

mu·cous

mu·cro *pl.* mu·cro·nes
    m. sterni

mu·cus

Mül·ler
    Charnley-M. total hip replacement
    M. arthrodesis
    M. hip prosthesis
    M. osteotomy
    M. plate
    M. procedure
    M. prosthesis
    M. total hip replacement

mul·ti·ar·tic·u·lar

mul·ti·zo·nal

Mum·ford
  M. procedure
  M. Gurd procedure

Münch·mey·er
  M's disease

MURCS as·so·ci·a·tion

Mur·phy
  M. sign
  M.-Lane bone skid
  Pierrot and M. procedure

Mur·ray
  Lucas and M. arthrodesis

mus·cle
  abdominal m's
  abductor m. of great toe
  abductor hallucis m.
  abductor m. of little finger
  abductor m. of little toe
  abductor m. of thumb,
    long
  abductor m. of thumb,
    short
  adductor m., great
  adductor m., long
  adductor m., short
  adductor m., smallest
  adductor m. of great toe
  adductor hallucis m.
  adductor m. of hip
  adductor m. of thigh
  adductor m. of thumb
  Albinus' m.
  anconeus m.
  anconeus m., lateral
  anconeus m., medial
  anconeus m., short
  appendicular m's
  articular m.
  articular m. of elbow
  articular m. of knee
  biceps m.
  biceps m. of arm
  biceps femoris m.
  biceps m. of thigh

mus·cle *(continued)*
  brachial m.
  brachioradial m.
  brachioradialis m.
  Chassaignac's axillary m.
  coccygeal m.
  coracobrachial m.
  coracobrachialis m.
  deltoid m.
  epitrochleoanconeus m.
  erector m. of spine
  extensor carpi radialis
    brevis m.
  extensor carpi radialis lon-
    gus m.
  extensor m. of digits, com-
    mon
  extensor m. of fingers
  extensor m. of fifth digit,
    proper
  extensor m. of great toe,
    long
  extensor m. of great toe,
    short
  extensor m. of index finger
  extensor m. of little finger
  extensor m. of thumb, long
  extensor m. of thumb,
    short
  extensor m. of toes, long
  extensor m. of toes, short
  external rotator m. of hip
  extrinsic m.
  extrinsic m. of foot
  femoral m.
  fibular m., long
  fibular m., short
  fibular m., third
  first palmar interosseous
    m.
  flexor m., accessory
  flexor m. of fingers, deep
  flexor m. of fingers, super-
    ficial
  flexor m. of great toe, long
  flexor m. of great toe,
    short

mus·cle *(continued)*

    flexor m. of little finger, short
    flexor m. of little toe, short
    flexor m. of thumb, long
    flexor m. of thumb, short
    flexor m. of toes, long
    flexor m. of toes, short
    flexor m. of wrist, radial
    flexor m. of wrist, ulnar
    gastrocnemius m.
    gastrocnemius m., lateral
    gastrocnemius m., medial
    gastrosoleus m.
    gemellus m., inferior
    gemellus m., superior
    gluteal m., least
    gluteus maximus m.
    gluteus minimus m.
    gracilis m.
    hamstring m's
    hypothenar m.
    iliac m.
    iliacus m.
    iliocostal m's
    iliopsoas m.
    infraspinatus m.
    infraspinous m.
    intercostal m.
    intercostal m's, external
    intercostal m's, innermost
    intercostal m's, internal
    internal rotator (hip) m.
    interossei m's of foot
    interosseous m's, palmar
    interosseous m's, plantar
    interosseous m's, volar
    interosseous m's of foot, dorsal
    interosseous m's of hand, dorsal
    interspinal m's
    interspinal m's of loins
    interspinal m's of neck
    interspinal m's of thorax
    intertransverse m's
    intertransverse m's, anterior

mus·cle *(continued)*

    intertransverse m's of neck, anterior
    intertransverse m's of neck
    intertransverse m's of thorax
    intrinsic m.
    intrinsic m. of foot
    Langer's m.
    lateral m. compartment of lower limb
    latissimus dorsi m.
    levator m's of ribs
    levator m's of ribs, long
    levator m's of ribs, short
    levator m. of scapula
    long m. of head
    long m. of neck
    longissimus m.
    longissimus m. of back
    longissimus colli m.
    longissimus m. of head
    longissimus m. of neck
    longissimus m. of thorax
    lumbrical m's of foot
    lumbrical m's of hand
    mesothenar m.
    multifidus m's
    m's of neck
    oblique m. of head, inferior
    oblique m. of head, superior
    obturator m., external
    obturator m., internal
    opposing m. of little finger
    opposing m. of thumb
    outer table m's
    palmar m., long
    palmar m., short
    paraspinal m's
    pectineal m.
    pectoral m., greater
    pectoral m., smaller
    peroneal m.
    peroneal m., long
    peroneal m., short

mus·cle *(continued)*

peroneal m., third
peroneus brevis m.
peroneus longus m.
peroneus tertius m.
pes anserinus m.
Phillips' m.
piriform m.
plantar m.
plantaris m.
popliteal m.
postaxial m.
posterior neck m.
preaxial m.
pretibial m's
pronator m., quadrate
pronator quadratus m.
pronator m., round
psoas m.
psoas m., greater
psoas m., smaller
quadrate m. of sole
quadrate m. of thigh
quadratus lumborum m.
quadriceps m.
quadriceps m. of thigh
rectus femoris m.
rhomboid m., greater
rhomboid m., lesser
rider's m's
rotator m's
rotator m's, long
rotator m's, short
rotator m. of hip
rotator m's of neck
rotator m's of thorax
sacrococcygeal m., anterior
sacrococcygeal m., dorsal
sacrococcygeal m., posterior
sacrococcygeal m., ventral
sacrospinal m.
sacrospinalis m.
sartorius m.
scalene m., anterior
scalene m., middle
scalene m., posterior
scalene m., smallest

mus·cle *(continued)*

scalenus m.
semimembranosus m.
semimembranous m.
semispinal m.
semispinal m. of head
semispinal m. of neck
semispinal m. of thorax
semitendinosus m.
semitendinous m.
serratus m., anterior
serratus m., posterior, inferior
serratus m., posterior, superior
skeletal m's
soleus m.
somatic m's
sphincter ani m.
spinal m.
splenius m. of head
splenius m. of neck
sternal m.
sternocleidomastoid m.
sternomastoid m.
strap m. of cervical spine
subclavius m.
subcostal m's
suboccipital m's
subscapular m.
subscapularis m.
supinator m.
supraspinatus m.
supraspinous m.
tensor m. of fascia lata
tensor fasciae latae m.
teres major m.
teres minor m.
thenar m's
tibial m., anterior
tibial m., posterior
trachelomastoid m.
transverse m. of thorax
transversospinal m.
trapezius m.
triceps m.
triceps m. of arm
triceps m. of calf

mus·cle *(continued)*
    vastus lateralis m.
    vastus medialis m.

mus·cu·lo·apo·neu·rot·ic

mus·cu·lo·skel·e·tal

mus·cu·lo·ten·di·nous

mus·cu·lus *pl.* mus·cu·li
    m. abductor digiti minimi manus
    m. abductor digiti minimi pedis
    m. abductor digiti quinti manus
    m. abductor digiti quinti pedis
    m. abductor hallucis
    m. abductor pollicis brevis
    m. abductor pollicis longus
    m. adductor brevis
    m. adductor hallucis
    m. adductor longus
    m. adductor magnus
    m. adductor minimus
    m. adductor pollicis
    m. anconeus
    m. articularis
    m. articularis cubiti
    m. articularis genu
    m. articularis genus
    m. biceps brachii
    m. biceps femoris
    m. brachialis
    m. brachioradialis
    musculi coccygei
    m. coccygeus
    musculi colli
    m. coracobrachialis
    m. deltoideus
    musculi dorsi
    m. epitrochleoanconaeus
    m. erector spinae
    m. extensor carpi radialis brevis
    m. extensor carpi radialis longus
    m. extensor carpi ulnaris

mus·cu·lus *(continued)*
    m. extensor digiti minimi
    m. extensor digiti quinti proprius
    m. extensor digitorum
    m. extensor digitorum brevis
    m. extensor digitorum communis
    m. extensor digitorum longus
    m. extensor hallucis brevis
    m. extensor hallucis longus
    m. extensor indicis
    m. extensor indicis proprius
    m. extensor pollicis brevis
    m. extensor pollicis longus
    musculi extremitatis inferioris
    musculi extremitatis superioris
    m. fibularis brevis
    m. fibularis longus
    m. fibularis tertius
    m. flexor accessorius
    m. flexor carpi radialis
    m. flexor carpi ulnaris
    m. flexor digiti minimi brevis manus
    m. flexor digiti minimi brevis pedis
    m. flexor digiti quinti brevis manus
    m. flexor digiti quinti brevis pedis
    m. flexor digitorum brevis
    m. flexor digitorum longus
    m. flexor digitorum profundus
    m. flexor digitorum sublimis
    m. flexor digitorum superficialis
    m. flexor hallucis brevis
    m. flexor hallucis longus
    m. flexor pollicis brevis

mus·cu·lus *(continued)*
   m. flexor pollicis longus
   m. gastrocnemius
   m. gemellus inferior
   m. gemellus superior
   m. gluteus maximus
   m. gluteus medius
   m. gluteus minimus
   m. gracilis
   m. iliacus
   m. iliocostalis
   m. iliocostalis cervicis
   m. iliocostalis dorsi
   m. iliocostalis lumborum
   m. iliocostalis thoracis
   m. iliopsoas
   m. infraspinatus
   musculi intercostales externi
   musculi intercostales interni
   musculi intercostales intimi
   musculi interossei dorsales manus
   musculi interossei dorsales pedis
   musculi interossei palmares
   musculi interossei plantares
   musculi interossei volares
   musculi interspinales
   musculi interspinales cervicis
   musculi interspinales lumborum
   musculi interspinales thoracis
   musculi intertransversarii
   musculi intertransversarii anteriores
   musculi intertransversarii anteriores cervicis
   musculi intertransversarii laterales
   musculi intertransversarii laterales lumborum

mus·cu·lus *(continued)*
   musculi intertransversarii mediales
   musculi intertransversarii mediales lumborum
   musculi intertransversarii posteriores
   musculi intertransversarii posteriores cervicis
   musculi intertransversarii thoracis
   m. latissimus dorsi
   musculi levatores costarum
   musculi levatores costarum breves
   musculi levatores costarum longi
   m. levator scapulae
   m. longissimus
   m. longissimus capitis
   m. longissimus cervicis
   m. longissimus dorsi
   m. longissimus thoracis
   m. longus capitis
   m. longus colli
   musculi lumbricales manus
   musculi lumbricales pedis
   musculi membri inferioris
   musculi membri superioris
   musculi multifidi
   m. obliquus capitis inferior
   m. obliquus capitis superior
   m. obturator externus
   m. obturator internus
   m. obturatorius externus
   m. obturatorius internus
   m. opponens digiti minimi
   m. opponens digiti quinti manus
   m. opponens pollicis
   m. palmaris brevis
   m. palmaris longus
   m. pectineus
   m. pectoralis major
   m. pectoralis minor

mus·cu·lus *(continued)*
   m. peroneus brevis
   m. peroneus longus
   m. peroneus tertius
   m. piriformis
   m. plantaris
   m. popliteus
   m. pronator quadratus
   m. pronator teres
   m. psoas major
   m. psoas minor
   m. quadratus femoris
   m. quadratus lumborum
   m. quadratus plantae
   m. quadriceps femoris
   m. rectus abdominis
   m. rectus capitis anterior
   m. rectus capitis lateralis
   m. rectus capitis posterior
    major
   m. rectus capitis posterior
    minor
   m. rectus femoris
   m. rhomboideus major
   m. rhomboideus minor
   musculi rotatores
   musculi rotatores breves
   musculi rotatores cervicis
   musculi rotatores longi
   musculi rotatores lum-
    borum
   musculi rotatores thoracis
   m. sacrococcygeus anterior
   m. sacrococcygeus dorsalis
   m. sacrococcygeus poste-
    rior
   m. sacrococcygeus ven-
    tralis
   m. sacrospinalis
   m. sartorius
   m. scalenus anterior
   m. scalenus medius
   m. scalenus minimus
   m. scalenus posterior
   m. semimembranosus
   m. semispinalis
   m. semispinalis capitis
   m. semispinalis cervicis

mus·cu·lus *(continued)*
   m. semispinalis dorsi
   m. semispinalis thoracis
   m. semitendinosus
   m. serratus anterior
   m. serratus posterior infe-
    rior
   m. serratus posterior supe-
    rior
   musculi skeleti
   m. soleus
   m. spinalis
   m. spinalis capitis
   m. spinalis cervicis
   m. spinalis dorsi
   m. spinalis thoracis
   m. splenius capitis
   m. splenius cervicis
   m. sternalis
   m. sternocleidomastoideus
   m. subclavius
   musculi subcostales
   musculi suboccipitales
   m. subscapularis
   m. supinator
   m. supraspinatus
   m. tensor fasciae latae
   m. teres major
   m. teres minor
   m. tibialis anterior
   m. tibialis posterior
   m. transversospinalis
   m. transversus thoracis
   m. trapezius
   m. triceps brachii
   m. triceps surae
   m. vastus intermedius
   m. vastus lateralis
   m. vastus medialis

Mus·tard
   M. iliopsoas transfer

my·al·gia
   m. cervicalis
   lumbar m.

My·a·pap Elix·ir

my·as·the·nia
 m. gravis

my·at·ro·phy

My·co·bac·te·ri·um
 M. tuberculosis

my·ec·to·my

my·ec·to·pia

my·ec·to·py

my·el·al·gia

my·el·ap·o·plexy

my·el·as·the·nia

my·el·ate·lia

my·el·at·ro·phy

my·el·auxe

my·el·en·ceph·a·li·tis

my·el·et·er·o·sis

my·elit·ic

my·eli·tis

my·elo·blas·to·ma

my·elo·cele

my·elo-CT

my·elo·cyst

my·elo·cys·to·cele

my·elo·cys·to·me·nin·go·
 cele

my·elo·cy·to·ma

my·elo·di·as·ta·sis

my·elo·dys·pla·sia

my·elo·en·ceph·a·li·tis

mye·elo·fi·bro·ma·to·sis

my·elo·fi·bro·sis
 osteosclerosis m.

my·elo·gram
 cisternal m.

my·elo·gram-CT

my·elog·ra·phy
 cervical m.
 lumbar m.
 metrizamide m.
 water-soluble m.

my·eloid

my·elo·ma
 multiple m.
 osteosclerotic m.
 plasma cell m.
 sclerosing m.

my·elo·ma·la·cia

my·elo·men·in·gi·tis

my·elo·me·nin·go·cele

my·elo·neu·ri·tis

my·elo·pa·ral·y·sis

my·elo·path·ic

my·elop·a·thy
 cervical m.
 external compressive m.

my·elo·phthi·sis

my·elo·ple·gia

my·elo·pro·lif·er·a·tive

my·elo·ra·dic·u·li·tis

my·elo·ra·dic·u·lop·a·thy

my·elor·rha·gia

mye·lor·rha·phy
 commissural m.

my·elo·scle·ro·sis

my·elo·syph·i·lis

my·elot·o·my

My·ers
 M. knee retractor

Myhre
 Ruvalcaba-M. syndrome

my·itis

myo·as·the·nia

myo·at·ro·phy

myo·blast

myo·blas·to·ma

myo·bra·dia

myo·cele

myo·ce·li·al·gia

myo·ce·li·tis

myo·cel·lu·li·tis

myo·ce·ro·sis

Myo·chry·sine

myo·cla·sis

myo·clon·ic

my·oc·lo·nus

myo·cyte

myo·cy·to·ma

myo·de·gen·er·a·tion

myo·de·mia

myo·di·as·ta·sis

my·odyn·ia

myo·dys·to·nia

myo·dys·tro·phia

myo·dys·tro·phy

myo·ede·ma

myo·fas·ci·tis

myo·fi·ber

myo·fi·bril

myo·fi·bril·la *pl.* myo·fi·bril·
   lae

myo·fi·bril·lar

myo·fi·bro·ma
   infantile m.

myo·fi·bro·sis

myo·fi·bro·si·tis

myo·fila·ment

My·o·flex

myo·ge·lo·sis

my·og·e·nous

myo·glo·bin·uria
   idiopathic m.

myo·hy·per·tro·phia
   m. kymoparalytica

my·oi·dem

my·oi·de·ma

myo·is·che·mia

myo·ke·ro·sis

myo·lem·ma

myo·li·po·ma

my·ol·y·sis

my·o·ma *pl.* my·o·mas, my·
   o·ma·ta

my·o·ma·la·cia

my·o·ma·tec·to·my

my·o·ma·to·sis

my·o·mec·to·my

myo·mel·a·no·sis

my·on

myo·ne·cro·sis
   clostridial m.

myo·neu·ral·gia

myo·neur·as·the·nia

myo·neu·rec·to·my

myo·neu·ro·ma

myo·neu·ro·sis

my·on·o·sus

myo·pa·chyn·sis

myo·pal·mus

myo·pa·ral·y·sis

myo·path·ia
    m. infraspinata

myo·path·ic

my·op·a·thy
    alcoholic m.
    centronuclear m.
    distal m.
    myotubular m.
    nemaline m.
    rod m.

myo·phage

my·oph·a·gism

myo·plasm

myo·plas·tic

myo·plas·ty

myo·psy·chop·a·thy

my·or·rha·phy

my·or·rhex·is

myo·sar·co·ma

myo·scle·ro·sis

myo·seism

myo·sit·ic

myo·si·tis
    m. a frigore
    m. fibrosa
    infectious m.
    interstitial m.
    multiple m.
    m. ossificans
    m. ossificans circumscripta
    m. ossificans progressiva
    m. ossificans traumatica

myo·si·tis *(continued)*
    parenchymatous m.
    progressive ossifying m.
    m. purulenta
    rheumatoid m.
    m. serosa

myo·spa·sia

myo·spasm

myo·spas·mia

myo·sta·sis

my·os·te·o·ma

myo·stro·ma

myo·su·ture

myo·syn·i·ze·sis

myo·ten·di·nous

myo·ten·on·to·plas·ty

myo·teno·si·tis

myo·te·not·o·my

myo·tome

myo·tom·ic

my·ot·o·my

myo·to·nia
    congenital m.

myo·troph·ic

my·ot·ro·phy

my·o·trop·ic

myxo·fi·bro·ma

myx·o·ma *pl.* myx·o·mas,
    myx·o·ma·ta

myxo·sar·co·ma

na·bu·ta·me·tone

Na·cha·mie
  Siffert-Foster-N. procedure

Nade
  N.-Rieth hip prosthesis

Naff·zig·er
  N. sign
  N. syndrome

Na·ger
  N. syndrome

nail
  Brooker-Wills n.
  Calandruccio n.
  cannulated n.
  cephalomedullary inter-
    locking n.
  cloverleaf n.
  Derby n.
  diagonal interlocking n.
  Ender n.
  femoral n.
  fused n.
  Gross-Kemph n.
  Hackenthall n.
  Hansen-Street n.
  Harris n.
  hippocratic n.
  Huckstep n.
  ingrown n.
  interlocking n.
  intramedullary n.
  Inyo n.
  Jewett n.
  Ken n.
  Ken sliding n.
  Klemm-Schellmann lock-
    ing n.
  Küntscher n.
  Lewis n.
  locked intramedullary n.
  locking Y n.
  Lottes n.

nail *(continued)*
  Massie n.
  nested n.
  Neufeld n.
  PGP n.
  Pugh n.
  reconstruction n.
  retrograde interlocking n.
  R-T (Russell-Taylor) re-
    construction n.
  Rush n.
  Russell-Taylor n.
  Rydell n.
  Schneider n.
  Seidel n.
  sliding n.
  Smillie n.
  Smith-Petersen n.
  Thornton n.
  tibial n.
  Uniflex n.
  Y-type interlocking n.
  Zickel n.

nail·ing
  elastic stable intramedul-
    lary n.
  exchange n.
  hip n.
  intramedullary n.
  marrow n.
  medullary n.
  reamed n.
  retrograde n.
  unreamed n.

nail start·er

Nale·buff
  N. arthrodesis
  N. deformity (Types I–V)

Nal·fon

Nam·a·qua·land
  N. hip dysplasia

NAON
    National Association of
    Orthopaedic Nurses

NAOT
    National Association of
    Orthopaedic Technolo-
    gists

α-naph·thol

Na·pro·syn

na·prox·en

nar·row·ing
    cartilage space n.
    disk space n.
    intervertebral space n.
    joint n.

Na·tion·al As·so·ci·a·tion of
Or·tho·pae·dic Nurs·es

Na·tion·al As·so·ci·a·tion of
Or·tho·pae·dic Tech·nol·o·
gists

Na·tion·al Board of Or·tho·
pae·dic Tech·nol·o·gists

Nau·ti·lus

na·vic·u·lar
    accessory n.

na·vic·u·lo·cap·i·tate

Nax·en

NBOT
    National Board of Ortho-
    paedic Technologists

Neal
    N.-Robertson litter

ne·ar·thro·sis

Neb·cin

neck
    anatomical n. of humerus
    n. of ankle bone
    false n. of humerus
    n. of femur

neck *(continued)*
    n. of fibula
    femoral n.
    n. of humerus
    lateral n. of vertebra
    n. of radius
    n. of rib
    n. of scapula
    scapular n.
    surgical n.
    surgical n. of humerus
    swan n.
    n. of talus
    true n. of humerus
    n. of vertebra
    n. of vertebral arch
    wry n.

ne·cro·sis *pl.* ne·cro·ses
    adiposytic n.
    aseptic n.
    avascular n.
    epiphyseal ischemic n.
    hyaline n.
    ischemic osteocytic n.
    superficial n.
    total n.

ne·crot·ic

nec·ro·tiz·ing

ne·crot·o·my
    osteoplastic n.

nee·dle
    Bunnell n.
    Keith n.
    spinal n.
    Tru-Cut n.

nee·dle hold·er
    Wangensteen n.h.

Nee·dles
    Melnick-N. syndrome

Neer
    Hassman, Brunn, and N.
     procedure
    N. capsular shift

Neer *(continued)*
    N. classification (for fractures of the proximal humerus)
    N. classification (for rotator cuff disease)
    N. lateral view
    N. prosthesis
    N. II total shoulder prosthesis
    N. transscapular view

Neis·se·ria
    N. gonorrhoeae

Né·la·ton
    N's dislocation
    N. line

Nel·son
    Janecki and N. procedure
    N. sign

neo·ar·thro·sis

Neo-Es·trone

Neo-Met·ric

neo·pla·sia
    intradural n.

neo·plasm
    musculoskeletal n.

neo·prene

Neo·sar

nerve
    axillary n.
    cervical n's
    cluneal n.
    common digital n.
    common peroneal n.
    cranial n's
    cutaneous n. of arm
    cutaneous n. of forearm
    cutaneous n. of hand
    deep peroneal n.
    digital n's
    digital n. of foot
    dorsal digital n.

nerve *(continued)*
    femoral n.
    n. hook
    lateral cutaneous n. of hand
    n. of Luschka
    median n.
    musculocutaneous n.
    obturator n.
    occipital n.
    peroneal n.
    phrenic n.
    pinched n.
    plantar n.
    posterior tibial n.
    pudendal n.
    radial n.
    saphenous n.
    sciatic n.
    sinuvertebral n.
    spinal n's
    spinal accessory n.
    superficial peroneal n.
    sural n.
    tibial n.
    ulnar n.
    vagus n.
    volar digital n.

Ner·vine

net·il·mi·cin

Ne·tro·my·cin

Neu
    N.-Laxova syndrome

Neu·feld
    N. nail
    N. roller traction

neu·ral·gia

neu·rar·throp·a·thy

neu·rec·to·my

neu·ri·tis
    idiopathic brachial n.

neu·ro·ar·throp·a·thy

Ninhydrin test

neu·ro·ca·nal

neu·ro·cen·tral

neu·ro·fi·bro·ma

neu·ro·fi·bro·ma·to·sis

neu·ro·fo·ra·men

neu·ro·gen·ic

neu·rol·y·sis

neu·ro·ma
    amputation n.
    Morton's n.
    traumatic n.

neu·ron
    motor n.
    sensory n.

neu·rop·a·thy
    peripheral n.

neu·ro·plas·ty

neu·ro·prax·ia

neu·ror·rha·phy

neu·ro·skel·e·ton

neu·ro·syph·i·lis

neu·ro·ten·sin

neu·rot·me·sis

neu·rot·o·my

neu·ro·trip·sy

Nev·i·as·er
    N. portal
    N. procedure

ne·vus *pl.* ne·vi

New·ing·ton
    N. orthosis

New Jer·sey knee pros·the·sis

New Jer·sey Low Con·tact
    Stress to·tal an·kle re·place·ment

New·ton
    N. ankle prosthesis
    N. total ankle replacement

New York cri·te·ria

New York Or·tho·pe·dic
    front-open·ing or·tho·sis

New York Uni·ver·si·ty in·sert

Nex·us To·tal Hip Sys·tem

Nich·o·las
    N. procedure

Ni·co·la
    N. procedure

Ni·cole
    Calnan-N. prosthesis

Ni·co·li
    N. graft

ni·dus *pl.* ni·di

Nie·bau·er
    N. implant
    N. prosthesis

Nie·mann
    N.-Pick disease

Nir·schl
    N. procedure

Nis·sen
    Brockman-N. arthrodesis

ni·tro·gen
    blood urea n. (BUN)

node
    Bouchard's n's
    gouty n.
    Haygarth's n's
    Heberden's n's
    Meynet's n's
    Schmorl's n.
    syphilitic n.

no·dos·i·ty
    Haygarth's n's

nod·u·lar

nod·ule
    Jeanselme's n's
    juxta-articular n's
    Lutz-Jeanselme n's
    Schmorl's n.

No·el
    Kramer, Craig, and N. os-
      teotomy

Noiles
    N. fully constrained device

no man's land

non·or·tho·pe·dic

non·seg·ment·ed

non·union
    juxta-articular n.

Noo·nan
    N's syndrome

Nor·gaard
    N. view

nor·mo·ten·sive

Nor·ris
    N. humeral extraction de-
      vice

Nor·ton
    N. ball reamer

no·tal·gia

notch
    acetabular n.
    clavicular n. of sternum
    coracoid n.
    costal n's of sternum
    cotyloid n.
    fibular n.
    greater sciatic n.
    interclavicular n.
    intercondylar n.
    intercondylar n. of femur
    intervertebral n.
    ischial n., greater
    ischial n., lesser

notch *(continued)*
    n. of ischium, greater
    n. of ischium, lesser
    jugular n. of sternum
    popliteal n.
    presternal n.
    radial n.
    radial n. of ulna
    sacrosciatic n., greater
    sacrosciatic n., lesser
    scapular n.
    sciatic n., greater
    sciatic n., lesser
    semilunar n. of scapula
    sternal n.
    suprascapular n.
    suprasternal n.
    trochlear n. of ulna
    ulnar n.
    ulnar n. of radius
    vertebral n., inferior
    vertebral n., superior

notch·plas·ty

No·vo Am·pi·cil·lin

No·vo·bu·ta·zone

No·vo·chlo·ro·cap

No·vo·ci·me·tine

No·vo·dox·yl·in

No·vo·lex·in

No·vo·meth·a·cin

No·vo·na·prox

No·vo·ni·da·zol

No·vo·pen-G

No·vo·pi·ro·cam

No·vo·pro·fen

No·vo-Sun·dac

No·vo·tet·ra

No·vo·tri·mel

Noyes
   N. test

NSAIA
   nonsteroidal anti-inflam-
      matory agent

NSAID
   nonsteroidal anti-inflam-
      matory drug

nu·cle·ot·o·my
   percutaneous n.

nu·cle·us *pl.* nu·clei
   n. gelatinosus
   n. pulposus
   n. pulposus disci interver-
      tebralis
   pulpy n.

Nu·prin

Nu-Tet·ra

Nys·trom
   Hessel/N. pin

NYU in·sert

O

OA
    occipitoatlantal
    osteoarthritis

OAWO
    opening abductory wedge
      osteotomy

Ober
    Inclan-O. procedure
    O's operation
    O. procedure
    O. test
    O.-Barr procedure

Ober·hill
    O. retractor

obliq·ui·ty
    o. of pelvis

obli·quus
    o. externus

O'Bri·en
    Fahey and O'B. procedure

ob·tu·ra·tor
    blunt o.
    cannula o.

oc·cip·i·tal·iza·tion

oc·cip·i·to·at·lan·tal

oc·ci·put

oc·clu·sion

oc·cult

Och·ro·my·cin V

ochro·no·sis

O'Con·nor
    O'C. finger dexterity test

oc·u·lo·hy·dro·ple·thys·mog·ra·phy

oc·u·lo·ple·thys·mog·ra·phy

oc·u·lo·pneu·mo·ple·thys·mog·ra·phy

Od·land
    O. ankle prosthesis

O'Don·o·ghue
    O'D. procedure

off·set
    humeral o.

Oga·nes·yan
    Volkov-O. fixation device

Og·den
    O. plate

Ogen

Og·ston
    O. line

Oh
    Froimson and O. proce-
      dure
    O. total hip replacement

OI
    osteogenesis imperfecta

olec·ra·nal

ole·cra·nar·thri·tis

ole·cra·nar·throp·a·thy

olec·ra·noid

olec·ra·non

olen·itis

oleo·chryso·ther·a·py

olis·the

olis·thy

Oli·ver
    Adams-O. syndrome

Ol·lier
    O's disease

Ol·lier *(continued)*
    O's law
    O. rake retractor
    O.-Thiersch skin graft

oma·gra

omal·gia

omar·thri·tis

omi·tis

Om·ni·fit ac·e·tab·u·lar cup

Om·ni·fit-HA fem·o·ral com·po·nent

Om·ni·fit To·tal Knee

Om·ni·paque

Om·ni·pen

omo·cla·vic·u·lar

omo·dyn·ia

omo·plata

omo·ster·num

One-Al·pha

on·kino·cele

on·y·chec·to·my

on·y·cho·cryp·to·sis

on·y·cho·my·co·sis

on·y·chot·o·my

open·ing
    o. in adductor magnus
      muscle
    o. of Hunter's canal, infe-
      rior
    o. of pelvis, inferior
    o. of pelvis, superior
    o. of sacral canal, inferior
    saphenous o.
    tendinous o.

op·er·a·tion (see also
    procedure and specific types
    of operation, such as
    arthroplasty)

op·er·a·tion *(continued)*
    Adams' o.
    Akin o.
    Albee's o.
    Albee-Delbet o.
    Albert's o.
    Alouette's o.
    Barker's o.
    Barsky's o.
    Barton's o.
    Berger's o.
    Bier's o.
    Buck's o.
    Chopart's o.
    Colonna's o.
    Dupuytren's o.
    flap o.
    Girdlestone o.
    Gritti's o.
    Guyon's o.
    Hancock's o.
    Hey's o.
    Hibbs' o.
    Hoffa's o.
    Hoffa-Lorenz o.
    Jaboulay's o.
    Keller o.
    Kocher's o.
    Lapidus o.
    Larrey's o.
    Lisfranc's o.
    Lorenz's o.
    McBride o.
    Mikulicz's o.
    Mitchell o.
    Ober's o.
    Péan's o.
    Phelps' o.
    Phemister o.
    Schede's o.
    Silver o.
    Steindler o.
    Stokes' o.
    Syme's o.
    Teale's o.
    Tikhor-Linberg o.
    Vladimiroff o.
    Whitman's o.

OPG
  oculoplethysmography

opis·the·nar

Opitz
  Smith-Lemli-O. syndrome

Op·pen·heim
  O. sign

op·po·nens
  o. bar
  o. digiti minimi
  o. digiti quinti
  o. pollicis

op·po·nens·plas·ty
  Brand o.
  Burkhalter o.
  Fowler o.
  Goldmar o.
  Groves o.
  Huber o.
  Littler o.
  Phalen-Miller o.
  Riordan o.

op·po·si·tion

Opti-Fix Hip Sys·tem

Oram
  Holt-O. syndrome

or·ange
  acid o. 10
  wool o. 2G

or·ce·in

Or·e·gon an·kle pros·the·sis

Or·e·gon Poly II an·kle pros·the·sis

Or·e·gon to·tal an·kle re·place·ment

or·ga·noph·i·lism

ORIF

Orr
  O. method
  O. technique

Orr *(continued)*
  O. treatment

or·the·sis *pl.* or·the·ses

or·thet·ic

or·thet·ics

or·the·tist

or·tho·dac·ty·lous

or·tho·dig·i·ta

or·thog·o·nal

or·tho·mel·ic

or·tho·pae·dic

or·tho·pae·dics

Or·tho·pae·dic Trau·ma As·so·ci·a·tion clas·si·fi·ca·tion (for tibial fracture stability)

or·tho·pe·dic

or·tho·pe·dics

or·tho·pe·dist

or·tho·pod

or·tho·prax·is

or·tho·praxy

or·tho·pros·the·sis

or·thor·rhach·ic

or·tho·sis *pl.* or·tho·ses
  A-frame o.
  abduction o. for hip
  ankle o.
  ankle-foot o.
  anterior control TLSO o.
  anteroposterior and medio-lateral control lumbosa-cral o.
  anteroposterior and medio-lateral control TLSO o.
  APR hip o.
  Boston o.

or·tho·sis *(continued)*
  cable twister o.
  Calcitite hip o.
  C.A.S.H. o.
  cervical o.
  cervicothoracolumbosacral
    o. (CTLSO)
  chairback o.
  clavicle o.
  dynamic knee o.
  elastic o.
  elastic twister o.
  elbow o.
  elbow-wrist-hand o.
  Engen extension o.
  Engen reciprocal o.
  flexible o.
  foot o.
  four-poster o.
  four-poster o. with exten-
    sion to waist
  Frejka o.
  functional o.
  Gillette o.
  hallux valgus o.
  hand o.
  hip o.
  hip-knee-ankle-foot o.
  hyperextension o.
  IRM spiral o.
  Jewett o.
  Klenzak o.
  knee o.
  knee-ankle-foot o.
  Knight-Taylor o.
  Lenox Hill o.
  long opponens o.
  lower limb o.
  lumbosacral o.
  Milwaukee o.
  Milwaukee cervicothora-
    columbosacral o.
  Newington o.
  New York Orthopedic
    front-opening o.
  overlapped upright for o.
  parapodium o.
  patellar tendon–bearing o.

or·tho·sis *(continued)*
  pillow o.
  plastic o.
  plastic floor reaction o.
  posterior and mediolateral
    control lumbosacral o.
  Profile hip o.
  PSA o.
  PTB o.
  Rancho o.
  rigid o.
  sacroiliac o.
  safety pin o.
  Saltiel o.
  Scottish Rite o.
  Seattle o.
  Shaeffer o.
  short opponens o.
  shoulder o.
  shoulder-elbow-wrist-
    hand o.
  SOMI o.
  spine o.
  spring wire o.
  standard ankle-foot o.
  standing frame o.
  static o.
  sternal occiput mandibular
    immobilization o.
  Tachdjian o.
  Taylor o.
  Teufel o.
  thermoplastic knee-ankle-
    foot o.
  thoracic o.
  thoraco-lumbar-sacral o.
    (TLSO)
  thoracolumbar o.
  thoracolumbosacral o.
  TIRR o.
  TLSO o.
  Toronto o.
  total-contact o.
  trilateral o.
  two-poster o.
  two-poster o. with exten-
    sion to waist
  UCB o.

or·tho·sis *(continued)*
    underarm o.
    upper limb o.
    Williams o.
    wrist-driven flexor
      hinge o.
    wrist-hand o.

Or·tho·Sorb pin

or·tho·ther·a·py

or·thot·ic

or·thot·ics

or·thot·ist
    certified o.

Or·tho·tron

Or·to·la·ni
    O's click
    O's sign

Oru·dis

os *pl.* os·sa
    o. acetabuli
    o. acromiale
    o. calcis
    o. capitatum
    o. carpale distale primum
    o. carpale distale quartum
    o. carpale distale secun-
      dum
    o. carpale distale tertium
    ossa carpalia
    ossa carpi
    o. centrale
    o. centrale tarsi
    o. coccygis
    o. costale
    o. coxae
    ossa cranialia
    o. cuboideum
    o. cuneiforme intermedium
    o. cuneiforme laterale
    o. cuneiforme mediale
    o. cuneiforme primum
    o. cuneiforme secundum
    o. cuneiforme tertium

os *(continued)*
    ossa digitorum manus
    ossa digitorum pedis
    o. femorale
    o. hamatum
    o. ilii
    o. ilium
    o. innominatum
    o. intercuneiforme
    o. intermedium
    o. intermetatarseum
    o. ischii
    o. lunatum
    o. magnum
    ossa membri inferioris
    ossa membri superioris
    ossa metacarpalia
    o. metacarpale tertium
    ossa metacarpi
    ossa metatarsalia
    ossa metatarsi
    o. multangulum majus
    o. multangulum minus
    o. naviculare
    o. naviculare manus
    o. naviculare pedis
    o. naviculare pedis retar-
      datum
    o. orbiculare
    o. pelvicum
    o. peroneum
    o. pisiforme
    o. pubis
    o. radiale
    o. sacrale
    o. sacrum
    o. scaphoideum
    o. sedentarium
    ossa sesamoidea manus
    ossa sesamoidea pedis
    o. subtibiale
    ossa suprasternalia
    ossa tarsalia
    o. tarsale distale primum
    o. tarsale distale quartum
    o. tarsale distale secun-
      dum
    o. tarsale distale tertium

os *(continued)*
    ossa tarsi
    o. tarsi fibulare
    o. tarsi tibiale
    ossa thoracis
    o. tibiale externum
    o. trapezium
    o. trapezoideum
    o. trigonum tarsi
    o. triquetrum
    o. vesalianum pedis

Os·borne
    O. and Cotterill procedure

Os·good
    O.-Schlatter disease
    O. osteotomy

Os·mond
    O.-Clarke procedure

os·phy·ar·thro·sis

os·sa

os·se·in

os·seo·apo·neu·rot·ic

os·seo·car·ti·lag·i·nous

os·seo·fi·brous

os·seo·in·te·gra·tion

os·seo·lig·a·ment·ous

os·seo·mu·cin

os·seo·mu·coid

os·se·ous

os·si·cle
    episternal o's
    intercalcar o's

os·sic·u·lar

os·si·des·mo·sis

os·sif·er·ous

os·sif·ic

os·si·fi·ca·tion
    cartilaginous o.

os·si·fi·ca·tion *(continued)*
    decreased o.
    ectopic o.
    endochondral o.
    heterotopic o.
    intramembranous o.
    perichondral o.
    periosteal o.

os·si·fied

os·tem·py·e·sis

os·sif·lu·ence

os·si·fy

os·si·fy·ing

os·sim·e·ter
    Küntscher o.

os·tal·gia

os·tar·thri·tis

os·te·al·gia

os·te·ana·bro·sis

os·te·ana·gen·e·sis

os·te·anaph·y·sis

os·te·ar·thri·tis

os·te·ar·throt·o·my

os·tec·to·my
    partial o.

os·te·ec·to·my

os·te·ec·to·pia

os·te·ec·to·py

os·te·in

os·te·ite

os·te·it·ic

os·te·itis
    acute o.
    o. albuminosa
    carious o.
    o. carnosa
    caseous o.

os·te·itis *(continued)*
  central o.
  chronic o.
  chronic nonsuppurative o.
  o. condensans
  o. condensans generalisata
  o. condensans ilii
  condensing o.
  condensing o. of clavicle
  cortical o.
  o. deformans
  fibrocystic o.
  o. fibrosa circumscripta
  o. fibrosa cystica
  o. fibrosa cystica general-
    isata
  o. fibrosa disseminata
  o. fibrosa localisata
  o. fibrosa osteoplastica
  formative o.
  o. fragilitans
  o. fungosa
  Garré's o.
  o. granulosa
  gummatous o.
  hematogenous o.
  multifocal o. fibrosa
  necrotic o.
  o. ossificans
  pagetoid o.
  parathyroid o.
  polycystic o.
  productive o.
  o. pubis
  rarefying o.
  sclerosing o.
  secondary hyperplastic o.
  o. tuberculosa cystica
  o. tuberculosa multiplex
    cystoides
  vascular o.

os·tem·py·e·sis

os·teo·ana·gen·e·sis

os·teo·an·es·the·sia

os·teo·an·eu·rysm

os·teo·ar·threc·to·my

os·teo·ar·thrit·ic
  endemic o.

os·teo·ar·thri·tis
  o. deformans
  o. deformans endemica
  hyperplastic o.
  interphalangeal o.
  premature o.

os·teo·ar·throp·a·thy
  familial o. of fingers
  hypertrophic o.
  hypertrophic o., idiopathic
  hypertrophic o., primary
  hypertrophic pneumic o.
  hypertrophic pulmonary o.
  idiopathic hypertrophic o.
  paraneoplastic o.
  pneumogenic o.
  primary hypertrophic o.
  pulmonary o.
  pustulotic o.
  secondary hypertrophic o.
  tabetic o.

os·teo·ar·thro·sis
  o. juvenilis

os·teo·ar·throt·o·my

os·teo·ar·tic·u·lar

os·teo·blast

os·teo·blas·tic

os·teo·blas·to·ma

os·teo·ca·chec·tic

os·teo·ca·chex·ia

os·teo·cal·cin

os·teo·camp·sia

os·teo·camp·sis

os·teo·car·ti·lag·i·nous

os·teo·chon·dral

os·teo·chon·dri·tis
  adolescent o.
  calcaneal o.
  o. deformans juvenilis
  o. deformans juvenilis
    dorsi
  o. dissecans
  o. ischiopubica
  juvenile deforming meta-
    tarsophalangeal o.
  o. necroticans
  o. ossis metacarpi et meta-
    tarsi
  o. patellae
  syphilitic o.

os·teo·chon·dro·ar·throp·a·
  thy

os·teo·chon·dro·dys·pla·sia

os·teo·chon·dro·dys·tro·phia
  o. deformans

os·teo·chon·dro·dys·tro·phy
  familial o.

os·teo·chon·dro·fi·bro·ma

os·teo·chon·drol·y·sis

os·teo·chon·dro·ma
  epiarticular o.
  epiphyseal o.
  fibrosing o.
  intra-articular o.

os·teo·chon·dro·ma·to·sis
  Ollier's o.
  synovial o.

os·teo·chon·dro·myx·o·ma

os·teo·chon·dro·path·ia

os·teo·chon·drop·a·thy
  polyglucose (dextran) sul-
    fate–induced o.

os·teo·chon·dro·phyte

os·teo·chon·dro·sar·co·ma

os·teo·chon·dro·sis
  o. deformans tibiae

os·teo·chon·dro·sis *(continued)*
  o. dissecans

os·teo·chon·drous

os·teo·cla·sia

os·te·oc·la·sis

os·teo·clast
  Collin's o.

os·teo·clas·tic

os·teo·clas·to·ma

os·teo·clas·ty

os·teo·com·ma

os·teo·cope

os·teo·cop·ic

os·teo·cra·ni·um

os·teo·cys·to·ma

os·teo·cyte

os·teo·des·mo·sis

os·teo·di·as·ta·sis

os·te·odyn·ia

os·teo·dys·pla·sia

os·teo·dys·plas·ty
  o. of Melnick and Needles

os·teo·dys·tro·phia
  o. cystica
  o. fibrosa

os·teo·dys·tro·phy
  Albright's hereditary o.
  azotemic o.
  parathyroid o.
  renal o.

os·teo·ec·ta·sia
  familial o.

os·teo·ec·to·my

os·teo·en·chon·dro·ma

os·teo·epiph·y·sis

os·teo·fi·bro·chon·dro·sar·co·ma

os·teo·fi·bro·ma

os·teo·fi·bro·ma·to·sis
   cystic o.

os·teo·fi·bro·sis

os·teo·flu·o·ro·sis

os·teo·gen

os·teo·gen·e·sis
   endochondral o.
     o. imperfecta (OI)
     o. imperfecta, type I
     o. imperfecta, type II
     o. imperfecta congenita
     o. imperfecta cystica
   periosteal o.

os·teo·ge·net·ic

os·te·o·gen·ic

os·te·og·e·nous

os·te·og·e·ny

os·teo·gram

os·te·og·ra·phy

os·teo·ha·lis·ter·e·sis

os·teo·hy·per·troph·ic

os·te·oid

os·teo·in·duc·tion

os·teo·in·duc·tive

os·teo·lipo·chon·dro·ma

os·teo·li·po·ma

Os·teo·lite

os·teo·lith

os·teo·lo·gia

os·te·ol·o·gist

os·te·ol·o·gy

os·te·ol·y·sis
   central o.
   familial expansile o.
   focal o.
   massive o.
   posttraumatic o.

os·teo·lyt·ic

os·te·o·ma
   osteoid o.

os·teo·ma·la·cia
   antacid-induced o.
   anticonvulsant o.
   familial hypophosphatemic
     o.
   hepatic o.
   infantile o.
   juvenile o.
   osteogenic o.
   puerperal o.
   renal tubular o.
   senile o.

os·teo·ma·la·cic

os·teo·mal·a·co·sis

os·teo·ma·to·sis

os·teo·mere

os·teo·meso·pyk·no·sis

os·teo·mi·o·sis

os·teo·my·elit·ic

os·teo·my·eli·tis
   acute o.
   chronic o.
   chronic hemorrhagic o.
   chronic sclerosing o.
   fungal o.
   diffuse sclerosing o.
   focal sclerosing o.
   Garré's o.
   hematogenous o.
   iatrogenic o.
   nonsuppurative o.
   pyogenic o.
   pyogenic vertebral o.

os·teo·my·eli·tis *(continued)*
   salmonella o.
   sclerosing nonsuppurative
     o.
   spinal m.
   tuberculous spinal o.
   suppurative o.
   typhoid o.
   vertebral o.
   o. variolosa

os·teo·my·elo·dys·pla·sia

os·teo·my·elog·ra·phy

os·teo·my·elo·scle·ro·sis

os·te·on

os·te·one

os·teo·ne·cro·sis
   traumatic o.

os·teo·nec·tin

Os·te·on·ics-HA fem·o·ral
im·plant

Os·te·on·ics to·tal hip re·
place·ment

os·teo·neu·ral·gia

os·te·on·o·sus

os·teo·path·ia
   o. condensans
   o. condensans disseminata
   o. condensans generalisata
   o. hemorrhagica infantum
   o. hyperostotica congenita
   o. hyperostotica multiplex
     infantilis
   o. striata

os·teo·path·ic

os·teo·pa·thol·o·gy

os·te·op·a·thy
   disseminated condensing
     o.
   myelogenic o.
   scorbutic o.

os·te·op·a·thy *(continued)*
   starvation o.

os·teo·pe·cil·ia

os·teo·pe·nia
   hyperthyroid o.

os·teo·pen·ic

os·teo·peri·os·te·al

os·teo·peri·os·ti·tis

os·teo·pe·tro·sis
   autosomal recessive–
     lethal o.

os·teo·phage

os·teo·phle·bi·tis

os·teo·phy·ma

os·teo·phyte
   bridging o's
   claw o.
   dorsal o.
   marginal o.
   marginal o. formation

os·teo·phy·to·sis
   spinal o.
   subperiosteal o.

os·teo·plaque

os·teo·pla·sia

os·teo·plast

os·teo·plas·tic

os·teo·plas·ti·ca

os·teo·plas·ty

os·teo·poi·ki·lo·sis

os·teo·poi·ki·lot·ic

os·teo·po·ro·sis
   o. of disuse
   idiopathic o.
   juvenile o.
   post-traumatic o.
   senile o.

os·teo·po·rot·ic

os·te·op·sath·y·ro·sis
  o. idiopathica

os·teo·ra·dio·ne·cro·sis

os·te·or·rha·gia

os·te·or·rha·phy

os·teo·sar·co·ma
  classical o.
  conventional o.
  dedifferentiated
    parosteal o.
  epithelioid o.
  gnathic o.
  high-grade surface o.
  idiopathic o.
  juxtacortical o.
  low-grade central o.
  multicentric o.
  multifocal o.
  parosteal o.
  periosteal o.
  primary o.
  secondary o.
  small-cell o.
  telangiectatic o.

os·teo·sar·co·ma·tous

Os·teo·scan-HDP

os·teo·scle·ro·sis
  o. congenita
  o. fragilis
  o. fragilis generalisata
  o. myelofibrosis

os·teo·scle·rot·ic

os·te·o·sis
  o. eburnisans monomelica
  ivory o.
  parathyroid o.
  renal o.

os·teo·spon·gi·o·ma

os·teo·su·ture

os·teo·syn·o·vi·tis

os·teo·syn·the·sis

os·teo·ta·bes

os·teo·te·lan·gi·ec·ta·sia

os·teo·throm·bo·phle·bi·tis

os·teo·throm·bo·sis

os·teo·tome
  box o.
  curved o.
  Hibbs o.
  Meyerding o.
  Smith-Petersen o.
  straight o.

os·te·ot·o·my
  Abbott and Gill o.
  acromion o.
  Amspacher and Messen-
    baugh o.
  Amstutz and Wilson o.
  angulation o.
  anteromedial displacement
    o.
  Bailey and Dubow o.
  Baker and Hill o.
  ball-and-socket o.
  Bellemore and Barrett o.
  block o.
  Blount o.
  Blount displacement o.
  Blundell Jones hip o.
  Blundell Jones varus o.
  Borden, Spencer, and
    Herndon o.
  Borggreve-van Ness rota-
    tion o.
  Brackett o.
  Brett o.
  Campbell tibial o.
  chevron o.
  Chiari o.
  closed-wedge o.
  closing abductory wedge o.
  Cole o.
  Cotton tibial o.
  Coventry o.
  Crego o.
  cuneiform o.

os·te·ot·o·my *(continued)*
  cup-and-ball o.
  cylindrical o.
  delta phalanx o.
  derotation o.
  dial o.
  Dickson o.
  Dimon o.
  displacement o.
  dome o.
  dorsal V o.
  dorsal wedge o.
  Dwyer o.
  Ferguson-Thompson o.
  Fish o.
  flexion o.
  French o.
  Gant o.
  Ghormley o.
  Haas o.
  high tibial o.
  hinge o.
  o. of hip
  Ingram o.
  innominate o.
  intertrochanteric o.
  Irwin o.
  Japas o.
  Kramer, Craig, and
    Noel o.
  Langenskiöld o.
  linear o.
  Lloyd-Roberts o.
  Lorenz's o.
  Lucas and Cottrell o.
  Macewen and Shands o.
  Macewen's o.
  Maquet o.
  Martin o.
  McCarroll o.
  McMurray o.
  Mitchell's o.
  Moore o.
  Müller o.
  opening abductory
    wedge o.
  opening-wedge o.
  open-wedge o.

os·te·ot·o·my *(continued)*
  Osgood o.
  Pauwels o.
  Pauwels-Y o.
  pelvic o.
  Pemberton o.
  phalangeal o.
  Phemister o.
  Platou o.
  Pott tibial o.
  proximal tibial o.
  radiohumeral o.
  rotational o.
  Salter o.
  Sarmiento o.
  Schanz o.
  Schede o.
  Sofield o.
  Southwick o.
  Speed o.
  spike o.
  steel-triradiate hip o.
  step o.
  step-down o.
  subtrochanteric o.
  Sugiuka o.
  Sutherland-Greenfield o.
  Thompson telescoping
    V o.
  tibial o.
  transtrochanteric o.
  valgus o.
  varus o.
  Whitman o.
  Y-o.

os·teo·tribe

os·teo·trip·sy

os·teo·trite

os·te·ot·ro·phy

os·te·ot·y·lus

os·ti·tis

Os·to·forte

os·to·sis

os·tot·o·my
    radioulnar rotational o.

os·tra·co·sis

OTR
    registered occupational
        therapist

Ot·to
    O's disease
    O. pelvis

out·let
    pelvic o.

out·rig·ger

over·drill

over·load
    axial compression o.
    facet o.

over·ream

over·rid·ing

over·toe

Over·ton
    O. lumbar spinal fusion

ox·al·ism

ox·ford
    orthopedic o.

Ox·ford knee pros·the·sis

Ox·ford uni·com·part·men·
    tal ar·thro·plas·ty

Ox·ford uni·com·part·men·
    tal de·vice

oxy·tet·ra·cy·cline

P/3
  proximal third

PA
  posteroanterior

P-A-C

pachy·dac·tyl·ia

pachy·dac·ty·ly

pachy·der·mo·peri·os·to·sis

pachy·onych·ia

pachy·peri·os·ti·tis

Pack
  P. amputation

pack
  cold p.
  hot p.

pack·ing

pad
  ABD p.
  abdominal p.
  calcaneal spur p.
  dinner p.
  distal p. for prosthesis
  fat p.
  Gelfoam p.
  heel p.
  infrapatellar fat p.
  knuckle p's
  metatarsal p.
  navicular p.
  patellar p.
  retropatellar fat p.
  scaphoid p.
  valgus knee control p.
  varus knee control p.

pad·ding
  cast p.
  felt p.

Pad·du
  P. procedure

Pa·get
  P. disease
  P's quiet necrosis

pa·get·ic

pain
  anterior knee p.
  bone p.
  diffuse back p.
  end stem p.
  inflammatory neck p.
  jumping p.
  localized p.
  low back p.
  mechanical p.
  nonradicular p.
  osteocopic p.
  patellofemoral p.
  phantom p.
  psychogenic p.
  radicular p.
  referred p.
  rest p.
  sclerotomal p.
  segmental p.
  spinal cord p.
  spondylogenic p.

pal·li·a·tive

Pal·lis·ter
  P.-Hall syndrome

palm
  handball p.

pal·mae

pal·mar

pal·mar·is
  p. longus

pal·pate

pal·pa·tion

pal·pi·ta·tion

pal·sy
    backpack p.
    Bell's p.
    cerebral p.
    Erb's p.
    handlebar p.
    high ulnar nerve p.

Pal·tri·ni·eri
    P. arthroplasty
    P.-Trentani resurfacing
      procedure

Pam·brin-IB

Pa·na·dol

pan·ar·te·ri·tis
    p. nodosa

pan·ar·thri·tis

Pan·ex

Pan·my·cin

Pan·ner
    P's disease

pan·nic·u·li·tis
    LE p.
    lupus p.

pan·nus

pan·os·te·itis

pan·os·ti·tis

Pan·to·paque

pan·tra·pe·zi·al

Pap·pas
    Buechel-P. total ankle re-
      placement

pap·ule
    painful piezogenic pedal
      p's
    piezogenic p's

para-ar·tic·u·lar

para·cen·te·sis

para·cnem·is

para·cne·mid·i·on

para·cox·al·gia

para·fuch·sin
    basic p.

para·lat·er·al

par·al·lag·ma

par·al·lel

pa·ral·y·sis *pl.* pa·ral·y·ses
    p. agitans
    Erb's p.
    familial periodic p.
    myopathic p.
    pseudohypertrophic mus-
      cular p.

para·me·ni·sci·tis

para·me·nis·cus

para·pa·re·sis

para·ple·gia

para·ple·gic

par·apoph·y·sis

para·rec·tus

para·sa·cral

para·scap·u·lar

para·spi·nal

para·ster·nal

para·syno·vi·tis

para·tar·si·um

para·ten·on

para·to·nia

para·ver·te·bral

pa·re·sis

par·es·the·sia

Par·ham
    P. band

Par·ker
  Bard-P. knife

Par·kin·son
  P's disease

Park·ridge
  Thompson, P., and Richards total ankle replacement

par·onych·ia
  p. tendinosa

par·os·te·al

par·os·te·itis

par·os·te·o·sis

par·os·ti·tis

par·os·to·sis

pars *pl.* par·tes
  p. abdominalis musculi pectoralis majoris
  p. annularis vaginae fibrosae digitorum manus
  p. annularis vaginae fibrosae digitorum pedis
  p. calcaneocuboidea ligamenti bifurcati
  p. calcaneonavicularis ligamenti bifurcati
  p. cartilaginea systematis skeletalis
  p. clavicularis musculi pectoralis majoris
  p. cruciformis vaginae fibrosae digitorum manus
  p. cruciformis vaginae fibrosae digitorum pedis
  p. iliaca lineae terminalis
  p. interarticularis
  p. lateralis arcus longitudinalis pedis
  p. lateralis musculorum intertransversariorum posteriorum cervicis
  p. lateralis ossis sacri
  p. libera membri inferioris

pars *(continued)*
  p. libera membri superioris
  p. medialis arcus longitudinalis pedis
  p. medialis musculorum intertransversariorum posteriorum cervicis
  p. ossea systematis skeletalis
  p. sacralis lineae terminalis
  p. sternocostalis musculi pectoralis majoris
  p. tibiocalcanea ligamenti medialis
  p. tibiocalcaneus ligamenti medialis
  p. tibionavicularis ligamenti medialis
  p. tibiotalaris anterior ligamenti medialis
  p. tibiotalaris posterior ligamenti medialis

Par·son·age
  P.-Turner syndrome

part
  broad p. of anterior annular ligament of leg
  lambdoidal (lower) p. of anterior annular ligament of leg
  superior p. of anterior annular ligament of leg
  third p. of quadriceps femoris muscle
  transverse p. of anterior annular ligament of leg

Par·tridge
  P. band
  P. cerclene system

Par·vin
  P. maneuver

pas·ser
  suture p.

pas·ser *(continued)*
    Swanson tendon p.
    tendon p.

pa·tel·la
    p. alta
    p. baja
    p. bipartita
    bipartite p.
    p. cubiti
    floating p.
    high-riding p.
    hypoplastic p.
    low-riding p.
    medial facet of p.
    p. partita
    slipping p.
    subluxation of p.
    subluxing p.
    tripartite p.

pa·tel·lar

pa·tel·lar clunk

pat·el·lec·to·my
    partial p.

pa·tel·lo·fem·o·ral

pat·en·cy

pat·ent

patho·me·chan·ics

Pat·rick
    P. maneuver
    P. test

pat·ten

pat·tern
    capsular p.
    instability p.
    onion-skin p.
    sunburst p.
    trabecular p.

pat·ty
    cottonoid p.

pau·ci·ar·tic·u·lar

Paul
    P's treatment

Paul·os
    P. procedure

Pau·wels
    P. angle
    P. osteotomy
    P.-Y osteotomy

pa·vil·ion
    p. of the pelvis

Pav·lik
    P. harness

Payr
    P. sign

PBG
    pedobarograph

PCA ac·e·tab·u·lar com·po·nent

PCA Po·rous-Coat·ed Hip

PCA to·tal hip re·place·ment

PCA un·con·strained de·vice

PCA uni·com·part·men·tal de·vice

PCE
    physical capacities evaluation

PCE (Smith)
    Smith physical capacities evaluation

PCL
    posterior cruciate ligament

PDS su·ture

pearl
    gouty p.

Pear·son
    P's attachment

pechy·agra

pec·ten *pl.* pec·ti·nes
    p. ossis pubis

pec·tin·e·al

pec·to·ral·gia

pec·to·ra·lis
    p. minor

pec·tus *pl.* pec·to·ra
    p. carinatum
    p. excavatum
    p. gallinatum
    p. recurvatum

ped·al

pe·dar·throc·a·ce

pe·des

Pe·dia·Pro·fen

ped·i·cle
    vascular p.
    p. of vertebral arch

pe·dic·u·lus *pl.* pe·dic·u·li
    p. arcus vertebrae

pedi·pha·lanx

pe·do·baro·graph
    dynamic p.

pe·do·graph

pe·dor·thic

pe·dor·thics

pe·dor·thist

Peel
    Blackburne and P. index

peg
    fixation p.

peg·board
    Purdue p.

Pel
    pelvic amputation

pel·lag·ra

Pel·le·gri·ni
    P.-Stieda disease

pel·vic

pel·vi·fem·o·ral

pel·vis *pl.* pel·ves, pelvises
    assimilation p.
    beaked p.
    bony p.
    coxalgic p.
    dwarf p.
    false p.
    flat p.
    greater p.
    high-assimilation p.
    kyphoscoliotic p.
    large p.
    lesser p.
    lordotic p.
    low-assimilation p.
    p. major
    p. minor
    p. nana
    p. ossea
    osteomalacic p.
    Otto p.
    p. plana
    Prague p.
    pseudo-osteomalacic p.
    rachitic p.
    Robert's p.
    Rokitansky's p.
    scoliotic p.
    small p.
    p. spinosa
    spondylolisthetic p.
    p. spuria
    true p.

pel·vi·sa·cral

pel·vi·sa·crum

pel·vi·ster·num

pel·vi·tro·chan·te·ri·an

pel·vo·spon·dy·li·tis
    p. ossificans

Pem·ber·ton
  P. osteotomy

Pe·na
  P.-Shokeir phenotype

Pen·brit·in

pen·cil
  electrosurgical p.

Pen·field
  P. dissector
  P. elevator

pen·i·cil·la·mine

pen·i·cil·lin

Penn·syl·va·nia Hip pros·
  the·sis

pen·ta·dac·tyl

Pen·tids

Pep·tol

per·ar·tic·u·la·tion

per·fo·rans *pl.* per·fo·ran·tes
  p. manus

peri·ac·e·tab·u·lar

peri·ar·thric

peri·ar·thri·tis
  calcific p.
  p. of shoulder

peri·ar·tic·u·lar

peri·bur·sal

peri·chon·dri·al

peri·chon·dri·tis

peri·chon·dri·um

peri·cox·itis

peri·des·mic

peri·des·mi·tis

peri·des·mi·um

peri·lu·nate

peri·my·elis

peri·my·eli·tis

peri·myo·si·tis

peri·mys·ia

peri·mys·i·al

peri·mys·i·itis

peri·mys·itis

peri·mys·i·um *pl.* peri·mys·
  ia
    external p.
    p. externum
    internal p.
    p. internum

peri·ost

peri·os·te·al

peri·os·te·itis

peri·os·teo·de·ma

peri·os·teo·ede·ma

peri·os·te·o·ma

peri·os·teo·med·ul·li·tis

peri·os·teo·my·eli·tis

peri·os·teo·phyte

peri·os·teo·sis

peri·os·teo·tome

peri·os·te·ot·o·my

peri·os·te·ous

peri·os·te·um

peri·os·ti·tis
    p. albuminosa
    albuminous p.
    diffuse p.
    hemorrhagic p.
    p. hyperplastica
    precocious p.

peri·os·to·ma

peri·os·to·med·ul·li·tis

peri·os·to·my

peri·os·to·sis

peri·os·tos·te·itis

peri·os·to·tome

peri·os·tot·o·my

peri·pa·tel·lar

pe·riph·er·al

peri·pros·thet·ic

peri·scle·ri·um

peri·spon·dyl·ic

peri·spon·dy·li·tis
    Gibney's p.

peri·sy·no·vi·al

peri·ten·din·e·um

peri·ten·di·ni·tis
    adhesive p.
    p. calcarea
    calcific p.
    p. crepitans
    p. serosa

peri·ten·di·nous

peri·te·non

peri·ten·o·ne·um

peri·ten·o·ni·tis

peri·ten·on·ti·tis

peri·to·ne·um

peri·tro·chan·ter·ic

peri·ver·te·bral

per·me·ative

pe·ro·nar·thro·sis

per·o·ne

per·o·ne·al

pe·ro·neo·tib·i·al

pe·ro·ne·us
    p. brevis
    p. longus
    p. tertius

per·os·se·ous

Per·ry
    P. procedure

Per·thes
    Legg-Calvé-P. disease
    P. disease

pes *pl.* pe·des
    p. abductus
    p. adductus
    p. anserinus
    p. calcaneocavus
    p. calcaneovalgus
    p. calcaneus
    p. cavus
    p. cavovalgus
    p. cavovarus
    congenital convex p. val-
      gus
    convex p. valgus
    p. curvus congenitus
    p. equinovalgus
    equinovarus p.
    p. gigas
    p. planovalgus
    p. planus
    p. pronatus
    p. supinatus
    p. valgus
    p. varus

pet·al·ing

pe·te·chiae

pe·te·chi·al

Pe·ter·sen
    Chuinard and P. arthro-
      desis

Pet·ries
    P. spica cast

PFC Mod·u·lar To·tal Knee
    Sys·tem

PFC To·tal Hip Sys·tem

Pfeif·fer
P's syndrome

PFFD
proximal femoral focal deficiency
proximal focal femoral deficiency

Pfi·zer·pen

P/3 fracture

PGDF
platelet-derived growth factor

PGP nail

Ph
phalangeal amputation

pha·lan·ge·al

pha·lan·gec·to·my
intermediate p.

pha·lan·ges

phal·an·gette
drop p.

phal·an·gi·tis

phal·an·gi·za·tion

pha·lan·go·pha·lan·ge·al

pha·lanx *pl.* pha·lan·ges
distal p.
phalanges digitorum manus
phalanges digitorum pedis
p. distalis digitorum manus
p. distalis digitorum pedis
phalanges of fingers
p. media digitorum manus
p. media digitorum pedis
middle p.
p. prima digitorum manus
p. prima digitorum pedis
proximal p.

pha·lanx *(continued)*
p. proximalis digitorum manus
p. proximalis digitorum pedis
p. secunda digitorum manus
p. secunda digitorum pedis
p. tertia digitorum manus
p. tertia digitorum pedis
phalanges of toes
ungual p. of fingers
ungual p. of toes

Pha·len
P. maneuver
P's sign
P. test
P.-Miller opponensplasty

phase
freezing p.
frozen p.
stance p.
swing p.
terminal stance p.
thawing p.

Pheas·ant
P. spacer

Phelps
P. procedure

Phem·is·ter
P. bone graft
P. graft
P. osteotomy

Phen·a·phen

phe·nol·iza·tion

phe·nom·e·non *pl.* phe·nom·e·na
cogwheel p.
halisteresis p.
Raynaud's p.
Rust's p.
staircase p.
tibial p.

phe·no·type
  Pena-Shokeir p.

phen·yl·bu·ta·zone

Phen·yl·one Plus

Phil·lips
  P. screw

phle·bit·ic

phle·bi·tis

phlebo·gram

phlebo·rhe·og·ra·phy
  venous p.

phlebo·throm·bo·sis

pho·co·me·lia
  complete p.
  distal p.
  proximal p.

Phoe·nix to·tal hip re·place·ment

pho·no·pho·re·sis

phos·pha·tase
  serum alkaline p.

phos·pha·ti·dyl·in·o·si·tol

phos·pha·ti·dyl·ser·ine

phos·pho·cre·a·tine

phos·pho·lip·id

phos·pho·mo·lyb·dic acid

phos·pho·pro·tein

phos·pho·rus
  inorganic p.

Phos·pho·tec

phos·pho·tung·stic acid

pho·to·ple·thys·mog·ra·phy

phys·e·al

phys·iat·rist

phys·i·ol·o·gy
  bone p.

phy·sis

Pick
  Niemann-P. disease

Pied·mont
  P. fracture

Pier·rot
  P. and Murphy procedure

pi·las·ter
  p. of Broca

pil·lar
  articular p.

Pil·li·ar
  P. total hip replacement

pil·lion
  p. fracture

pil·low
  abduction p.
  IMP-Capello slimline abduction p.

pin
  absorbable p.
  clavicle p.
  p. cutter
  femoral guide p.
  Gouffon p.
  guide p.
  Hagie p.
  halo p.
  Hessel/Nystrom p.
  Knowles p.
  Lottes p.
  medullary p.
  Moore p.
  OrthoSorb p.
  Rush p.
  skeletal traction p.
  Steinmann p.
  Street medullary p.
  suture p.
  threaded p.
  threaded Steinmann p.

pinch
    key p.
    pulp p.

Pio·trow·ski
    P. sign

PIP
    proximal interphalangeal

pip·er·a·cil·lin

PIP fu·sion

Pip·ra·cil

Pi·ro·goff
    P. amputation
    P. stump

pir·ox·i·cam

pit
    costal p.

piv·ot

plane
    anatomic p.
    anteroposterior p.
    auricular p. of sacral bone
    coronal p.
    fascial p.
    frontal p.
    Hensen's p.
    horizontal p.
    longitudinal p.
    median p.
    midsagittal p.
    popliteal p. of femur
    sagittal p.
    sternal p.
    transverse p.
    vertical p.

pla·no·val·gus

plan·ta pe·dis

plan·tal·gia

plan·tar

plan·ta·ris

pla·num *pl.* pla·na

pla·num *(continued)*
    p. popliteum femoris
    p. sternale

plaque
    attachment p's

Pla·que·nil

plas·ma
    fresh frozen p.

plas·ma·cy·to·ma
    solitary p.

Plas·ta·zote col·lar

plas·ter
    Minerva p.
    p. of Paris

plas·tic·i·ty

plas·ti·sol

plas·tron

plas·ty
    T-p.
    V-Y p.
    Z-p.

plate
    Alta titanium reconstruc-
       tion p.
    anchor p.
    angled p.
    angled compression p.
    AO p.
    Bagby compression p.
    blade p.
    Blount p.
    bone p.
    buttress p.
    compression p.
    cribriform p.
    dynamic compression p.
    Eggers p.
    Eggers bone p.
    Elliott p.
    Elliott femoral condyle
       blade p.
    end p.

plate *(continued)*
   epiphyseal p.
   femoral p.
   femoral condyle blade p.
   femur p.
   p. fixation
   foot p.
   growth p.
   heavy side p.
   Lane p's
   low-profile p.
   McLaughlin p.
   metal foot p.
   Moe p.
   Moe intertrochanteric p.
   Moore p.
   Müller p.
   nail p.
   Ogden p.
   one-third semitubular p.
   one-third tubular p.
   overlay p.
   Roy-Camille p.
   Sherman p.
   side p.
   slide p.
   soft-tissue p.
   Steffee p.
   subchondral p.
   Townley tibial plateau p.
   volar p.
   Whitman p.
   Wilson p.
   Yuan p.
   Yuan I p.
   Zimmer femoral condyle
     blade p.
   Zuelzer hook p.

pla·teau
   tibial p.

plate·let

plat·ing

Platt
   Putti-P. procedure

platy·ba·sia

platy·cne·mia

platy·cne·mic

platy·kne·mia

platy·me·ria

platy·me·ric

platy·po·dia

pla·tys·ma

platy·spon·dyl·ia

platy·spon·dyl·i·sis

platy·spon·dy·ly

pled·get

pleo·mor·phic

ple·on·os·te·o·sis
   Leri's p.

ple·thys·mo·graph
   impedance p.

ple·thys·mog·ra·phy

pleu·ra·poph·y·sis

pleu·ro·cen·trum

plex·op·a·thy
   brachial p.

plex·us *pl.* plex·us, plex·us·es
   brachial p.
   cervical p.
   lumbar p.
   sciatic p.

pli·ca *pl.* pli·cae
   plicae alares
   infrapatellar p.
   lateral p.
   lateral suprapatellar p.
   medial suprapatellar p.
   mediopatellar p.
   suprapatellar p.
   synovial plicae
   p. synovialis
   p. synovialis infrapatel-
     laris

pli·ca *(continued)*
    p. synovialis mediopatel-
      laris
    p. synovialis patellaris
    p. synovialis suprapatel-
      laris

pli·ers
    needle-nosed p.

PLIF
    posterolateral interbody
      fusion

Plt
    platelets

plug
    bicorticate p.
    bone p.
    tricorticate p.

PMMA
    polymethyl methacrylate

PMS Me·tro·ni·da·zole

PMS Sul·fa·sal·a·zine

pneu·mar·thro·sis

pneu·mo·arth·ro·gram

PO_4
    phosphate

po·dag·ra

pod·a·gral

po·dag·ric

pod·a·grous

po·dal·gia

pod·ar·thri·tis

pod·ede·ma

point
    glenoid p.
    ossification p.
    ossification p., primary
    ossification p., secondary
    trigger p.

point·er
    hip p.
    shoulder p.

POL
    posterior oblique ligament

Po·land
    P. anomaly
    P. moment of inertia
    P. syndrome

po·lio·my·eli·tis

pol·lex *pl.* pol·li·ces
    p. extensus
    p. flexus
    p. valgus
    p. varus

pol·lic·i·za·tion
    Buck-Gramko p.
    Gillies p.
    Littler p.
    Riordan p.
    Verdan p.

Pol·lock
    P. amputation

poly·ac·e·tyl

poly·ac·rylo·ni·trile

poly·ar·ter·itis
    p. nodosa

poly·ar·thral·gia
    p.-arthritis

poly·ar·thric

poly·ar·thrit·ic

poly·ar·thri·tis
    benign p.
    chronic osteolytic p.
    chronic secondary p.
    chronic villous p.
    p. destruens
    infectious p.
    peripheral p.
    rheumatoid p.
    symmetric p.

poly·ar·thri·tis *(continued)*
    tuberculous p.
    vertebral p.
    xanthomatous p.

pol·y·ar·tic·u·lar

poly·cen·tric

Poly·cen·tric un·con·strained de·vice

Poly·cil·lin

poly·dac·ty·ly
    central p.
    radial p.
    revision p.
    short rib–p., Majewski type
    short rib–p., non-Majewski type
    ulnar p.

Poly-Di·al in·sert sys·tem

poly·di·ox·an·one

poly·dys·spon·dy·lism

poly·eth·y·lene
    high-density p.
    ultrahigh molecular weight p. (UHMWPE)

poly·glac·tin 910

poly·gly·col·ic acid
    braided p.a.

poly·meta·car·pia

poly·meta·tar·sia

poly·meth·acry·late

poly·meth·yl
    p. methacrylate

poly·my·op·a·thy

poly·myo·si·tis

poly·neu·rit·ic

poly·neu·ri·tis

poly·os·tot·ic

pol·yp

poly·peri·os·ti·tis
    p. hyperesthetica

poly·pro·py·lene
    braided p.

poly·syn·o·vi·tis

poly·ten·di·ni·tis

poly·ten·di·no·bur·si·tis

poly·teno·syn·o·vi·tis

poly·tet·ra·flu·o·ro·eth·y·lene

Pon·cet
    P's disease
    P's rheumatism

pop·les

pop·lit·e·al

poro·coat·ing

po·ro·sis

po·rot·ic

po·rous-coat·ed

por·tal
    Neviaser p.

Por·te·noy
    P's classification

po·si·tion
    anatomic p.
    barber-chair p.
    bayonet p.
    beach-chair p.
    Bonner's p.
    Brickner p.
    p. of fracture fragment
    frog-leg p.
    Jones' p.
    open p.
    proximal bow p.
    reverse Trendelenburg p.
    semi-Fowler p.

po·si·tion·er
    cup p.
    McGuire pelvic p.

post
    thumb p.

post·ax·i·al

post·bra·chi·al

post·cu·bi·tal

Pos·tel
    D'Aubigne-P. Scale (for
      hip replacement results)

pos·ter·i·or

post·fib·u·lar

post·is·chi·al

pos·ture
    benediction p.

po·tas·si·um

po·ten·tial
    piezoelectric p.
    streaming p.
    stress-generated p.
    zeta p.

Pott
    P's disease
    P. tibial osteotomy

Pot·ter
    P. arthrodesis

pouch
    suprapatellar p.

Pou·part
    P. inguinal ligament

Pow·er
    P's ratio

PPD
    purified protein derivative

PPG
    photoplethysmography

PPi
    pyrophosphate

Pra·der
    P.-Willi syndrome

pre·ax·i·al

Pre·cef

Pre·ci·sion Hip

Pre·ci·sion Os·teo·block Hip

pre·cos·tal

pre·hal·lux

pre·hen·sion

Prei·ser
    P's disease

Prem·a·rin

Pren·yl jac·ket

pre·odon·toid

prep
    lupus erythematosus p.
      (LE prep)

pre·pa·tel·lar

pre·scap·u·la

pre·scap·u·lar

pre·spon·dy·lo·lis·the·sis

Press-fit Con·dy·lar Mod·u·
lar To·tal Knee Sys·tem

pres·sure
    bone marrow p.
    intradiskal p.
    intraosseous p.
    p. sore

pre·ster·num

pre·swing

pre·zy·ga·poph·y·sis

PRG
    phleborheography

Pri·max·in

Prin·ci·pen

Pritch·ard
  P. elbow prosthesis
  P.-Walker elbow pros-
    thesis

pro·cal·lus

pro·ce·dure (see also *operation*
  and specific types of
  procedure, such as
  arthroplasty)
  Akin p.
  Albee shelf p.
  Amspacher and Messen-
    baugh p.
  Amstutz resurfacing p.
  Anderson p.
  Anderson and Hutchins p.
  Austin p.
  Baker p.
  Bankart p.
  Barr p.
  Barr-Record p.
  Batchelor-Brown p.
  Bateman p.
  Beckenbaugh p.
  Bentzon's p.
  Berman and Gartland p.
  B.H. Moore p.
  bicentric resurfacing p.
  Bleck p.
  Bosworth p.
  Bosworth shelf p.
  Boyd and Anderson p.
  Boyd and McLeod p.
  Boyd and Sisk p.
  Brahms p.
  Braun p.
  Brett p.
  Brett and Campbell p.
  Bristow p.
  Bristow-Latarjet p.
  Brittain p.
  Brockman p.
  Brooks and Saddon p.
  Brown p.
  Bugg and Boyd p.

pro·ce·dure *(continued)*
  Bunnell p.
  Caldwell and Durham p.
  Campbell p.
  Campbell and Akbarnia p.
  Carroll p.
  Cave and Rowe p.
  Chandler p.
  Chaves-Rapp p.
  Chiari shelf p.
  Cho p.
  Chrisman and Snook p.
  Clancy p.
  Cloward p.
  Codivilla p.
  Cole p.
  Coleman p.
  Colonna shelf p.
  Copeland and Howard p.
  Couch, DeRosa, and
    Throop p.
  coxa vara p.
  Cubbins p.
  Darrach p.
  Das Gupta p.
  D'Aubigne p.
  Debeyre p.
  Dewar and Barrington p.
  Dickson-Diveley p.
  Dimon and Hughston p.
  double cup p.
  Dunn p.
  Dunn-Brittain p.
  du Toit and Roux p.
  DuVries p.
  Dwyer p.
  Eden-Hybbinette p.
  Eden-Lange p.
  eggshell p.
  Ellis p.
  Ellis Jones p.
  Ellison p.
  Elmslie-Cholmeley p.
  Elmslie-Trillat p.
  Enneking p.
  L'Episcope Zachary p.
  Ericksson p.
  Essex-Lopresti p.

pro·ce·dure *(continued)*
    Evans p.
    Eyler p.
    Fahey and O'Brien p.
    Fairbanks and Sever p.
    Farmer p.
    Forbes p.
    Fowler p.
    Fowles p.
    Fox-Blazina p.
    Frank Dickson shelf p.
    Freeman resurfacing p.
    French p.
    Fried and Green p.
    Froimson and Oh p.
    Frost p.
    Fulkerson p.
    Gallis p.
    Garceau p.
    Gelman p.
    genu recurvatum p.
    Gerard resurfacing p.
    Getty spine p.
    Giannestras p.
    Gill p.
    Gill shelf p.
    Girdlestone-Taylor p.
    Graber-Duvernay p.
    Green p.
    Grice p.
    Grice-Green p.
    Gruca p.
    Hammon p.
    Hark p.
    Harmon p.
    Harris-Beath p.
    Hassman, Brunn, and
      Neer p.
    Hauser p.
    Heifetz p.
    Herndon-Heyman p.
    Hey-Groves shelf p.
    Heyman p.
    Heyman-Herndon p.
    Hibbs p.
    His-Haas p.
    Hitchcock p.
    Hodgson p.

pro·ce·dure *(continued)*
    Hoffer p.
    Hohmann p.
    Hoke p.
    Hovanian p.
    Hughston p.
    Hughston and Jacobson p.
    Inclan-Ober p.
    Indiana conservative re-
      surfacing p.
    Ingram p.
    Janecki and Nelson p.
    Japas p.
    Jones p.
    J.R. Moore p.
    Juvara p.
    Kapel p.
    Karakousis and
      Vezeridis p.
    Kaufer p.
    Keller p.
    Kendrick p.
    Kessler p.
    keyhole p.
    Kidner p.
    Kiehn-Earle-DesPrez p.
    Kortzeborn p.
    Krukenberg p.
    Lam modification of
      Jones p.
    Lambrinudi p.
    Lange p.
    Langenskiöld p.
    Lapidus p.
    Leeds p.
    Legg p.
    L'Episcope Zachary p.
    Lewis and Chekofsky p.
    Liebolt p.
    Lindeman p.
    Lindholm p.
    Lloyd-Roberts p.
    Localio p.
    Loose p.
    Losee p.
    Lowman p.
    Lowman shelf p.
    Luck p.

pro·ce·dure *(continued)*
   Ludloff p.
   Lynn p.
   McBride p.
   MacCarthy p.
   McCarty p.
   McCash p.
   McCauley p.
   McElvenny p.
   MacIntosh p.
   McKeever p.
   McLaughlin p.
   McReynolds p.
   Magnuson p.
   Magnuson-Stack p.
   Ma and Griffith p.
   Majestro, Ruda, and
     Frost p.
   Malawer p.
   Maquet p.
   Marcove, Lewis, and
     Horos p.
   Marshall p.
   Martin p.
   Mauck p.
   Mayo p.
   Menson and Scheck p.
   Milch p.
   Miller p.
   Mitchell p.
   Miyakawa p.
   B.H. Moore p.
   J.R. Moore p.
   Muller p.
   Mumford-Gurd p.
   Neviaser p.
   Nicholas p.
   Nicola p.
   Nirschl p.
   Ober p.
   Ober-Barr p.
   O'Donoghue p.
   Osborne and Cotterill p.
   Osmond-Clarke p.
   over-the-top p.
   Paddu p.
   Paltrinieri-Trentani resur-
     facing p.

pro·ce·dure *(continued)*
   Paulos p.
   Peabody p.
   Perry p.
   Phelps p.
   Pierrot and Murphy p.
   Putti p.
   Putti-Platt p.
   Radley, Liebig, and
     Brown p.
   Reichenheim-King p.
   resurfacing p.
   Reverdin-Green p.
   reverse Mauck p.
   Rose p.
   Roux-Goldthwait p.
   Ruiz-Moro p.
   Saha p.
   Saltzer resurfacing p.
   Sargent p.
   Sarmiento p.
   Schrock p.
   Scott p.
   Scudari p.
   Selig p.
   Sharrard-Trentani resur-
     facing p.
   shelf p.
   Siffert-Foster-Nachamie p.
   Silver p.
   Silfverskiöld p.
   Slocum p.
   Snow-Litler p.
   Southwick slide p.
   Soutter p.
   Speed p.
   Speed and Boyd p.
   Spira p.
   Spittler p.
   Staheli p.
   Stanisavljevic p.
   Staples-Black-Brostrom p.
   steel shelf p.
   Steindler p.
   Stener and Gunterberg p.
   Stewart p.
   Stone p.
   Strayer p.

pro·ce·dure *(continued)*

Suppan p.
Sutherland p.
Swanson p.
Thomas p.
Thomas, Thompson, and Straub p.
Tikhor-Linberg p.
Tillman resurfacing p.
Tohen p.
Trillat p.
Turco p.
Veleanu, Rosianu, and Ionescu p.
Vulpius p.
Vulpius-Compere p.
Wagner p.
Wagner resurfacing p.
Warner and Farber p.
Watson-Jones p.
Weaver and Dunn p.
West and Soto-Hall p.
White p.
White slide p.
Whitman p.
Whitman-Thompson p.
Wiberg shelf p.
Wilson p.
Wilson and Jacobs p.
Wilson and McKeever p.
Winograd p.
Wolf p.
Woodward p.
Young p.
Zadik p.
Zarins and Rowe p.
Zeir p.

pro·cess

accessory p. of sacrum, spurious
acromial p.
acromion p.
alar p. of sacrum
anconeal p. of ulna
articular p. of axis, anterior
articular p. of coccyx, false

pro·cess *(continued)*

articular p. of sacrum, spurious
ascending p's of vertebrae
calcaneal p. of cuboid bone
calcanean p.
calcanean p. of cuboid bone
capitular p.
condyloid p. of vertebrae, inferior
condyloid p. of vertebrae, superior
conoid p.
coracoid p.
coronoid p.
cubital p. of humerus
dentoid p. of axis
descending p's of vertebrae
ensiform p. of sternum
epiphyseal p.
falciform p. of rectus abdominis muscle
hamular p. of unciform bone
inframalleolar p. of calcaneus
intercondylar p. of tibia
internal p. of humerus
lateral p. of calcaneus
mamillary p's of sacrum, oblique
oblique p. of vertebrae, inferior
oblique p. of vertebrae, superior
odontoid p. of axis
olecranon p. of ulna
sacralized transverse p.
spinal p.
spinous p.
spinous p. of sacrum, spurious
spinous p. of tibia
Stieda's p.
styloid p.
styloid p. of fibula
styloid p. of radius

pro·cess *(continued)*
    styloid p. of ulna
    synovial p.
    transverse p.
    transverse p. of sacrum
    transverse p. of vertebrae,
        accessory
    trochlear p. of calcaneus
    unciform p. of scapula
    uncinate p. of unciform
        bone
    uncinate p's of vertebra
    ungual p. of third phalanx
        of foot

pro·ces·sus *pl.* pro·ces·sus
    p. accessorii spurii
    p. accessorius
    p. articularis inferior ver-
        tebrarum
    p. articularis superior os-
        sis sacri
    p. articularis superior ver-
        tebrarum
    p. calcaneus ossis cuboidei
    p. coracoideus scapulae
    p. coronoideus ulnae
    p. costalis vertebrae
    p. costarius vertebrae
    p. lateralis tali
    p. lateralis tuberis calca-
        nei
    p. mamillaris
    p. medialis tuberis calca-
        nei
    p. posterior tali
    p. spinosus vertebrarum
    p. styloideus fibulae
    p. styloideus ossis meta-
        carpalis III
    p. styloideus radii
    p. styloideus ulnae
    p. supracondylaris humeri
    p. supracondyloideus hu-
        meri
    p. transversus vertebra-
        rum
    p. trochlearis calcanei

pro·ces·sus *(continued)*
    p. xiphoideus

pro·chon·dral

pro·col·la·gen

pro·cur·va·tion

Pro·cy·tox

Pro·fen

Pro·file hip or·tho·sis

Pro·file To·tal Hip Sys·tem

Pro·gens

pro·gres·sion
    cross-legged p.
    curve p.

pro·jec·tion
    Ficat's p.
    Jacovsky's p.
    Laurin's p.
    Merchant's p.
    Settegast's p.

pro·lif·er·ate

pro·lif·er·a·tion
    villous lipomatous p.

pro·lif·er·a·tive

Pro·lo·prim

prom·on·to·ri·um *pl.* prom·
    on·to·ria
    p. ossis sacri

pro·na·tion

pro·na·tion-ab·duc·tion

pro·na·tion-aver·sion

pro·na·tion-dor·si·flex·ion

pro·na·to·flex·or

pro·na·tor
    p. quadratus
    p. teres

prone

pro·phy·lax·is

Pro·plast

pro·prio·cep·tion

pro·prio·cep·tive

pro·prio·cep·tor

pro·ster·na·tion

pros·the·sis *pl.* pros·the·ses
    above-knee p.
    acetabular p.
    acrylic p.
    AHSC elbow p.
    Anatomic Porous Replace-
        ment (APR) p.
    anatomic surface elbow p.
    ankle p.
    Anthropometric Total Hip
        (ATH) p.
    Arizona elbow p.
    Arizona Health Science
        Center–Volz elbow p.
    Austin-Moore hip p.
    Bahler elbow p.
    Bateman p.
    Bateman bipolar p.
    Bechtol p.
    below-knee p.
    BIAS total hip p.
    Biax wrist p.
    bicentric femoral head p.
    Biomet Total Toe p.
    Biometric p.
    bipolar p.
    bipolar femoral p.
    Blauth knee p.
    Botta p.
    Brigham knee p.
    Calnan-Nicole p.
    capitellocondylar elbow p.
    cemented p.
    cemented porous-coated p.
    Charnley's p.
    chromium cobalt p.
    Cofield p.
    collared p.
    collarless p.
    Compartmental II knee p.

pros·the·sis *(continued)*
    Conaxial ankle p.
    Conoidal ankle p.
    constrained p.
    Coonrad elbow p.
    custom-made p.
    D'Aubigne hip p.
    Dee elbow p.
    DePalma p.
    DF-80 hip p.
    digital p.
    Dubinet hip p.
    Eaton p.
    Eftekhar hip p.
    Eicher hip p.
    elbow p.
    Endo-Model p.
    Endo-Model rotating knee
        joint p.
    Ewald elbow p.
    femoral head p.
    Flatt p.
    Flatt finger/thumb p.
    Flatt metacarpophalangeal
        p.
    fully constrained knee p.
    geometric knee p.
    Gristina and Webb p.
    GSB elbow p.
    Gschwind, Scheir, and
        Bahler elbow p.
    GUEPAR knee p.
    Hamas p.
    Harris Precoat Plus P.
    Henschke-Mauch p.
    hinged p.
    hip p.
    humeral p.
    humeral head p.
    ICLH ankle p.
    ICLH elbow p.
    Indiana conservative p.
    Insall-Burstein p.
    internal p.
    Ishizuki elbow p.
    Kessler p.
    Kirschner II-C shoulder p.
    knee p.

pros·the·sis *(continued)*
  Kudo elbow p.
  Lewis expandable adjustable p.
  Link V p.
  Liverpool elbow p.
  London elbow p.
  Lowe-Miller elbow p.
  lower limb p.
  Lubinus SP II hip p.
  McBride hip p.
  McKee elbow p.
  McKee-Farrar p.
  McKeever p.
  Madreporic hip p.
  Mallory-Head p.
  manual locking of knee p.
  Matchett-Brown hip p.
  Mayo ankle p.
  Mayo elbow p.
  Mazas elbow p.
  metal on metal p.
  Meuli wrist p.
  Michael Reese p.
  Minns knee p.
  Mittlemeier hip p.
  modular p.
  Moore hip p.
  Morscher hip p.
  MOSC (Miami Orthopaedic Surgical Clinics) p.
  Mueller p.
  Naden-Rieth hip p.
  Neer p.
  Neer II total shoulder p.
  New Jersey knee p.
  Newton ankle p.
  Niebauer p.
  noncemented p.
  Odland ankle p.
  Oregon ankle p.
  Oregon Poly II ankle p.
  Oxford knee p.
  patellar p.
  Pennsylvania Hip p.
  plastic on metal p.
  pneumatic on-knee p.

pros·the·sis *(continued)*
  porous-coated p.
  posterior cruciate condylar p.
  posterior cruciate ligament-retaining p.
  posterior cruciate ligament-sacrificing p.
  posterior stabilized p.
  Precision Stem and Neck (PSN) p.
  Pritchard elbow p.
  Pritchard-Walker elbow p.
  provisional p.
  PTB-SC p.
  PTB-SC-SP p.
  PTB supracondylar suprapatellar p.
  radiocarpal flexible hinge p.
  Ring hip p.
  Roper-Tuke elbow p.
  Rothman Institute total hip p.
  safety on-knee p.
  St. George-Buchholz ankle p.
  Sbarbaro tibial plateau p.
  Scheier elbow p.
  Schlein elbow p.
  semiconstrained knee p.
  Smith ankle p.
  Souter elbow p.
  Spectron EF hip p.
  S-ROM femoral p.
  Stanmore elbow p.
  Steffee interphalangeal p.
  Steffee metacarpophalangeal p.
  Strickland metacarpophalangeal p.
  Swanson p.
  T-28 (Trapezoidal 28) p.
  Taperloc p.
  Taperloc hip p.
  tendon p.
  Thompson femoral head p.
  Thompson hip p.

pros·the·sis *(continued)*
    threaded titanium acetab-
        ular p. (TTAP)
    total hip p.
    TPR ankle p.
    Trapezoidal 28 (T-28) p.
    Tri-Axial elbow p.
    uncemented p.
    unconstrained p.
    unconstrained knee p.
    upper limb p.
    Valls hip p.
    Volz p.
    Wadsworth elbow p.
    Wagner p.
    Walldius knee p.
    wrist p.
    Zimmer shoulder p.
    Zweymuller hip p.

pros·thet·ic

pros·thet·ics

pros·the·tist
    certified p.

Prot
    protein

pro·tein
    bone morphogenetic p.
    bone morphogenic p.
    core p.
    C-reactive p.
    link p.
    S-100 p.
    total blood p.

pro·teo·gly·can

pro·teo·lip·id

Pro·te·us
    P. syndrome

pro·to·chon·dral

pro·to·chon·dri·um

pro·to·col·la·gen

Pro·to·stat

Pro-Trac cru·ci·ate re·con·
    struc·tion sys·tem

pro·trac·tor

Pro·trin

pro·tru·sio
    p. acetabuli

pro·tru·sion
    intrapelvic p.

prox·i·mal

proximal/3
    proximal third

pro·zo·nal

PSA or·tho·sis

pseud·an·ky·lo·sis

pseud·ar·thri·tis

pseud·ar·thro·sis
    interspinous p.

pseu·do·an·ky·lo·sis

pseu·do·ar·thri·tis

pseu·do·ar·thro·sis

pseu·do·cap·sule

pseu·do·clau·di·ca·tion

pseu·do·cox·al·gia

pseu·do·epiph·y·sis

pseu·do·frac·ture

pseu·do·gout

pseu·do·hy·po·para·thy·roi·
    dism

pseu·do·lux·a·tion

pseu·do·me·nin·go·cele

Pseu·do·mo·nas

pseu·do-os·teo·ma·la·cia

PSN (Precision Stem and
    Neck) pros·the·sis

pso·as

pso·itis

pso·ri·a·sis
   arthritic p.
   p. arthropathica
   p. arthopica

pso·ri·at·ic

psy·cho·mo·tor

PTA
   posttraumatic arthritis

PTB
   patellar tendon bearing

PTB or·tho·sis

PTB-SC (supracondylar) pros·the·sis

PTB-SC-SP (supracondylar suprapatellar) pros·the·sis

pter·nal·gia

PTFE
   polytetrafluoroethylene

PTH
   parathyroid hormone

PTLA
   percutaneous transluminal angioplasty

PTT
   partial thromboplastin time

pu·bi·ot·o·my

pu·bis pl. pu·bes

pu·bo·coc·cyg·e·al

pu·bo·fem·o·ral

pu·bo·tib·i·al

Pugh
   P. nail

Pu·gi·fix fist splint

pull

pul·ley
   p. of finger
   flexor p.

pulp
   digital p.

Pul·ver
   P.-Taft finger flexion

pump
   high-flow arthroscopy p.
   infusion p.

pump bump

punch
   cortical gauge p.
   gauge p.
   Kerrison p.
   Michele p.

punc·tate

punc·tum pl. punc·ta
   p. ossificationis
   p. ossificationis primarium
   p. ossificationis secundarium

punc·ture
   lumbar p.

Purdue
   P. pegboard

Pu·rine·thol

pur·pu·ra

Pur·ser
   Sharp-P. test

pu·ru·lent

push·er
   knot p.

Put·ti
   P. arthrodesis
   P. bone rasp
   P. procedure
   P. rasp
   P.-Platt procedure

PVO
pyogenic vertebral osteo-myelitis

PVR
pulse volume recorder

py·ar·thro·sis

pyk·no·dys·os·to·sis

Pyle
P. metaphyseal dysplasia

py·lon
adjustable p.

pyo·ar·thro·sis

pyo·gen·ic

PYP
pyrophosphate

py·ram·i·da·le

py·rex·ia *pl.* py·rex·iae

Py·ro·lite

py·ro·phos·phate
^{99m}Tc-labeled p.

py·ru·vate

Q an·gle

quad·ra·ti·pro·na·tor

quad·ra·tus
    q. plantaris

quad·ri·ceps·plas·ty
    V-Y q.

quad·ri·ple·gia
    average q.
    high q.
    low q.
    respirator-dependent q.

quad·ri·ple·gic

Quain
    triangular fascia of Q.

quar·ti·ster·nal

Queck·en·stedt
    Q. sign

Quen·gle
    Q. cast

Quer·vain
    Q's disease
    Q's fracture

Quick Pep

qui·es·cence

Quig·ley
    Meyn and Q. maneuver
    Q. traction

quin·ti·ster·nal

R
  radius, complete (congenital absence of limb)

r
  radius, incomplete (congenital absence of limb)

RA
  rheumatoid arthritis

RAAGG
  rheumatoid arthritis agglutination

RAAGG test

rab·bet·ting

ra·chi·al

ra·chi·al·gia

ra·chi·cen·te·sis

ra·chid·i·al

ra·chid·i·an

ra·chil·y·sis

ra·chio·camp·sis

ra·chio·chy·sis

ra·chio·cy·pho·sis

ra·chi·odyn·ia

ra·chio·ky·pho·sis

ra·chio·my·eli·tis

ra·chio·pa·ral·y·sis

ra·chi·op·a·thy

ra·chio·ple·gia

ra·chio·sco·li·o·sis

ra·chio·tome

ra·chi·ot·o·my

ra·chis

ra·chis·ag·ra

ra·chis·chi·sis

ra·chi·tis

ra·chit·o·my

rack
  Graft R.

ra·di·al

ra·di·a·lis

rad·i·cot·o·my

ra·dic·u·lec·to·my

ra·dic·u·li·tis
  cervical r.
  spinal r.
  unilateral r.

ra·dic·u·lo·neu·ri·tis

ra·dic·u·lop·a·thy
  unilateral r.

ra·dii

ra·dio·bi·cip·i·tal

ra·dio·cap·i·tate

ra·dio·cap·i·tel·lar

ra·dio·car·pal

ra·dio·car·pus

ra·dio·dig·i·tal

ra·dio·gram

ra·dio·graph
  frog-leg r.
  lateral flexion-estension r.
  skyline r.

ra·dio·graph·ic

ra·di·og·ra·phy

ra·dio·hu·mer·al

ra·di·ol·o·gist

ra·dio·lu·cen·cy

ra·dio·lu·cent

ra·dio·lun·ate

ra·di·opaque

ra·dio·scapho·cap·i·tate

ra·dio·scaph·oid

Ra·di·os·tol

ra·dio·ther·a·py

ra·dio·tri·que·tral

ra·dio·ul·nar

ra·di·us *pl.* ra·dii
   r. curvus

ra·dix *pl.* ra·di·ces
   r. arcus vertebrae

Rad·ley
   R., Liebig, and Brown approach
   R., Liebig, and Brown procedure

Rai·miste
   R. sign

RAM un·con·strained de·vice

ra·mus *pl.* ra·mi
   r. inferior ossis ischii
   r. inferior ossis pubis
   inferior r. of pubis
   inferior pubic r.
   r. of ischium
   r. ossis ischii
   r. ossis pubis
   pubic r.
   r. pubicus
   r. of pubis
   r. of pubis, ascending
   r. of pubis, descending
   superior pubic r.
   superior r. of pubis
   r. superior ossis ischii
   r. superior ossis pubis
   superior r. of pubis

Ran·a·wat
   R's method

Ran·cho
   R. orthosis

range
   r. of motion

ra·ni·ti·dine

ra·phe *pl.* ra·phae
   median r. of neck, posterior
   mental r.

Rapp
   Chaves-R. procedure

rar·e·fac·tion

RA slide
   rheumatoid arthritis slide test

rasp
   bone r.
   circle r.
   Fischer r.
   Putti r.
   Putti bone r.

ratch·et

rate
   erythrocyte sedimentation r.
   sedimentation r.

rat·ing
   Mazur ankle r.

ra·tio
   A/G r. (albumin/globulin)
   Blackburne r.
   calcar cortical r.
   Insall r.
   Insall-Salvati r.
   Poisson r.
   Power's r.

Rau·ber
   spinal crest of R.

ray
  digital r.
  metatarsal r's
  stiff r.

Ray·naud
  R's disease
  R's phenomenon
  R's sign

RBC
  red blood (cell) count

re·ab·sorb

re·ab·sorp·tion

re·ac·tion
  periosteal r.

read·ing
  wet r.

re·a·gent
  calcium buffer r.
  calcium-binding r.

re·align·ment
  tendon r.

ream·er
  acetabulum r.
  awl r.
  ball r.
  brace-type r.
  center core r.
  center-cutting r.
  Chandler r.
  conical r.
  cortical r.
  end-cutting r.
  hand r.
  handle-type r.
  Harris center-cutting r.
  head r.
  medullary canal r.
  Norton ball r.
  Rush awl r.
  spiral r.
  spiral cortical r.
  spiral trochanteric r.
  taper r.

ream·er *(continued)*
  T-handled r.
  trochanteric r.

ream·ing
  eccentric r.

re·bal·anc·ing
  tendon r.

re·cess
  accessory r. of elbow
  acetabular r.
  inferior r.
  sacciform r. of articulation
    of elbow
  superior r.

re·ces·sus *pl.* re·ces·sus
  r. sacciformis articula-
    tionis cubiti
  r. sacciformis articula-
    tionis radioulnaris dis-
    talis
  r. subpopliteus

Reck·ling·haus·en
  R's disease of bone

re·con·struc·tion
  capsular r.
  post axial polydactyly r.

Re·cord
  Barr-R. procedure

re·cord·er
  pulse volume r.

re·cov·ery
  spinal root r.

re·cruit·ment
  fiber r.

rec·tus
  r. abdominis
  r. femoris

re·cur·va·tum

red
  basic r. 9
  natural r. 28

re·dis·lo·ca·tion

Red·lund
    R.-Johnell method

re·duc·er
    Fiske & SubbaRow r.

re·duc·tion
    closed r.
    closed hip r.
    Crego hip r.
    Ferguson r.
    r. of fracture
    Howorth r.
    Lange r.
    Lorenz r.
    open r.
    open hip r.
    open r. and internal fixa-
      tion
    Ridlon hip r.
    Scaglietti r.
    Somerville hip r.

Reed
    R.-Sternberg cells

reef·ing

re·flex
    Achilles r.
    Babinski's r.
    biceps r.
    Chaddock r.
    Mendel-Bekhterev r.
    Moro's r.
    nuchocephalic r.
    quadriceps r.
    sympathetic dystrophy r.
    tendon r.
    triceps r.

re·frac·ture

re·gio *pl.* re·gi·o·nes
    r. calcanea
    r. dorsalis manus
    r. dorsalis pedis
    r. plantaris pedis

rehab
    rehabilitation

re·ha·bil·i·tate

re·ha·bil·i·ta·tion

Rei·chen·heim
    R.-King procedure

re·im·plan·ta·tion
    delayed r.
    one-stage r.
    primary exchange r.
    two-stage r.

Rei·ter
    R's syndrome

Rel·a·fen
    rebound r.

re·lax·ant
    muscle r.

re·lax·a·tion

re·lease
    abductor pollicis longus r.
    acrosyndactyly r.
    arthroscopic retinacular r.
    capsular r.
    carpal tunnel r.
    de Quervain r.
    Fowler r.
    lateral retinacular r.
    tendon r.
    wrist r.

re·lux·a·tion

re·mod·el·ing
    bone r.
    regressive r.

re·pair
    arthroscopic r.
    Bankart r.
    boutonnière r.
    Bunnell tendon r.
    five-in-one r.
    Kessler tendon r.
    Kleinert tendon r.
    triad knee r.

re·pair *(continued)*
   Tsuge tendon r.
   Verdan tendon r.

re·place·ment
   Alvine total ankle r.
   Amstutz total hip r.
   Averill total hip r.
   Biofit total hip r.
   bipolar total hip r.
   Buechel-Pappas total
     ankle r.
   cementless total hip r.
   Charnley-Müller total
     hip r.
   CHD total hip r.
   Christiansen total hip r.
   Contour DF-80 total hip r.
   Engh total hip r.
   Exeter total hip r.
   Freeman total hip r.
   Giliberty total hip r.
   Harris total hip r.
   Harris-Galante total hip r.
   Hastings total hip r.
   HD 2 total hip r.
   Howse total hip r.
   Iowa total hip r.
   Jaffee total hip r.
   joint r.
   Judet total hip r.
   Ling total hip r.
   Lord total hip r.
   Lunceford total hip r.
   McKee-Farrar total hip r.
   Madreporic total hip r.
   Matchett-Brown total
     hip r.
   Mayo total ankle r.
   Monk total hip r.
   Müller total hip r.
   New Jersey Low Contact
     Stress total ankle r.
   Newton total ankle r.
   Oh total hip r.
   Oregon total ankle r.
   Osteonics total hip r.
   PCA total hip r.

re·place·ment *(continued)*
   Phoenix total hip r.
   Pilliar total hip r.
   polycentric total knee r.
   porous-coated total hip r.
   press-fit total hip r.
   Ring total hip r.
   Ring UPM total hip r.
   Sarmiento total hip r.
   Scarborough total hip r.
   self-bearing ceramic total
     hip r.
   Sivash total hip r.
   Smith total ankle r.
   Stanmore total hip r.
   STH-2 total hip r.
   T-28 total hip r.
   Takahura total ankle r.
   Thompson, Parkridge, and
     Richards total ankle r.
   total ankle r.
   total condylar knee r.
   total hip r.
   total joint r.
   TPL-6 total hip r.
   Trapezoidal total hip r.
   tricompartmental r. of
     knee
   unicompartmental r. of
     knee
   University of California,
     Irvine, total ankle r.
   Varikopf total hip r.
   Wilson-Burstein total
     hip r.

re·plan·ta·tion

re·sec·tion
   bone r.
   distal clavicle r.
   Girdlestone r.
   panmetatarsal head r.
   pedicle r.
   ray r.
   rib r.
   talar dome r.
   vertebral body r.

re·sec·tor
  full-radius r.
  synovial r.

re·sid·u·al

re·sorp·tion
  bone r.
  idiopathic r.

re·sponse
  loading r.

rest
  notochordal r.

re·sur·fac·ing
  patellar r.

re·tic·u·lo·cy·to·sis
  cerebroside r.

re·tic·u·lo·en·do·the·li·o·ma
  lipid r.

re·tic·u·lo·his·ti·o·cy·to·ma

re·tic·u·lo·his·ti·o·cy·to·sis
  multicentric r.

re·tic·u·lum *pl.* re·tic·u·la
  sarcoplasmic r.

ret·i·nac·u·lum *pl.* ret·i·nac·u·la
  r. of arcuate ligament
  r. capsulae articularis
    coxae
  contracted lateral r.
  r. costae ultimae
  digital r.
  dorsal r.
  extensor r.
  extensor r. of foot, inferior
  extensor r. of foot, superior
  extensor r. of hand
  r. extensorum manus
  flexor r. of foot
  flexor r. of hand
  r. flexorum manus
  r. ligamenti arcuati

ret·i·nac·u·lum *(continued)*
  r. musculorum extensorum
    pedis inferius
  r. musculorum extensorum
    pedis superius
  r. musculorum fibularium
    inferius
  r. musculorum fibularium
    superius
  r. musculorum flexorum
    pedis
  r. musculorum peronaeo-
    rum inferius
  r. musculorum peronaeo-
    rum superius
  r. musculorum peroneo-
    rum inferius
  r. musculorum peroneo-
    rum superius
  r. patellae laterale
  r. patellae mediale
  patellar r., lateral
  patellar r., medial
  peroneal r., inferior
  peroneal r., superior
  sixth compartment r.
  r. tendinum
  r. tendinum musculorum
    extensorum
  r. tendinum musculorum
    extensorum inferius
  r. tendinum musculorum
    extensorum superius
  r. tendinum musculorum
    flexorum
  Weitbrecht's r.

re·trac·tion
  disk-space r.

re·trac·tor
  Adson cerebellum r.
  Adson-Beckman r.
  Adson-Beckwith r.
  Army r.
  Balfour r.
  Beckman r.
  Bennett r.
  Blount knee r.

re·trac·tor *(continued)*
    cerebellum r.
    Chandler r.
    Cloward self-retaining r.
    cobra r.
    double end r.
    Downing r.
    Hibbs r.
    Hohman r.
    Holscher root r.
    Israel r.
    knee r.
    malleable r.
    Markham Meyerding r.
    Mayo-Collins r.
    Meyerding's r.
    Myers knee r.
    Oberhill r.
    Ollier rake r.
    patella r.
    pin r.
    Richardson r.
    Scoville r.
    self-retaining r.
    Senn double end r.
    Smillie r.
    Sofield r.
    stay r.
    Steinmann pin r.
    Taylor r.
    Thompson r.
    U.S. r.
    Volkmann rake r.
    Weitlaner r.

re·trad

retriever
    suture r.

ret·ro·cal·ca·neo·bur·si·tis

ret·ro·col·lis

ret·ro·cru·ral

ret·ro·grade

ret·ro·lis·the·sis

ret·ro·lis·thet·ic

ret·ro·pulsed

ret·ro·pul·sion
    bony r.

ret·ro·spon·dy·lo·lis·the·sis

ret·ro·tor·sion

ret·ro·ver·sion

re·vas·cu·lar·iza·tion

Re·ver·din
    R.-Green procedure
    R. skin graft

Re·verse Ratch·et rod

re·vi·sion
    amputation r.
    hip r.
    joint r.
    Marks and Bayne r.
    stump r.
    swan-neck r.

Re·za·i·an
    R. fixation device
    R. spinal fixator

RF
    rheumatoid factor

rhab·do·my·ol·y·sis
    exertional r.

rhab·do·myo·sar·co·ma

rhae·bo·cra·nia

rhae·bo·sce·lia

rhae·bo·sis

rhe·os·to·sis

rheu·mar·thri·tis

rheu·ma·tal·gia

rheu·mat·ic

rheu·ma·tism
    apoplectic r.
    articular r., chronic
    Besnier's r.
    Heberden's r.

rheu·ma·tism *(continued)*
    lumbar r.
    MacLeod's capsular r.
    muscular r.
    nodose r.
    osseous r.
    palindromic r.
    Poncet's r.
    subacute r.
    tuberculous r.
    visceral r.

rheu·ma·tis·mal

rheu·ma·to·gen·ic

rheu·ma·toid

rheu·ma·tol·o·gist

rheu·ma·tol·o·gy

rheu·ma·to·sis

Rheu·ma·trex

rhi·zo·mel·ic

rhi·zot·o·my

Rho·dis

rhom·boi·de·us
    r. major
    r. minor

rib
    abdominal r's
    r. approximator
    bicipital r.
    bifid r.
    r. contractor
    cervical r.
    false r's
    floating r's
    r. raspatory
    rudimentary r.
    r. shears
    slipping r.
    spurious r's
    sternal r's
    sternebral r.
    Stiller's r.
    true r's

rib *(continued)*
    vertebral r's
    vertebrochondral r's
    vertebrocostal r's
    vertebrosternal r's

rib-belt

Ri·card
    R's amputation

Rich·ards
    R. button
    Thompson, Parkridge, and
        R. total ankle replace-
        ment

Ri·chard·son
    R. retractor

rick·ets
    adult r.
    anticonvulsant r.
    pseudo–vitamin D defi-
        ciency r.
    vitamin D–dependent r.
    vitamin D–refractory r.
    vitamin D–resistant r.
    X-linked hypophospha-
        temic r.

Ri·dau·ra

ridge
    bicipital r., anterior
    bicipital r., external
    bicipital r., internal
    bicipital r., outer
    bicipital r., posterior
    deltoid r.
    epicondylic r., lateral
    epicondylic r., medial
    gastrocnemial r.
    gluteal r. of femur
    r. of humerus
    interarticular r. of head of
        rib
    interosseous r. of fibula
    interosseous r. of radius
    interosseous r. of tibia
    interosseous r. of ulna

ridge *(continued)*
    intertrochanteric r.
    middle r. of femur
    r. of neck of rib
    oblique r's of scapula
    pectoral r.
    radial r. of wrist
    rough r. of femur
    supinator r.
    supracondylar r. of hu-
      merus, lateral
    supracondylar r. of hu-
      merus, medial
    transverse r's of sacrum
    trapezoid r.
    tubercular r. of sacrum
    ulnar r. of wrist
    vastus lateralis r.

Rid·lon
    R. hip reduction

Rieth
    Nade-R. hip prosthesis

ri·gid·i·ty
    torsional r.

ri·gid·us

Ri·ley
    Robinson and R. spinal fu-
      sion
    R.-Day syndrome

rim
    glenoid r.

Ring
    R. curette
    R. hip prosthesis
    R. total hip replacement
    R. unconstrained device
    R. UPM total hip replace-
      ment

ring
    cricoid r.
    drop-lock r.
    fibrous r., interpubic
    fibrous r. of intervertebral
      disk

ring *(continued)*
    locking r.
    Mose concentric r.
    periosteal bone r.
    thumb r.

Ri·or·dan
    Haddad-R. arthrodesis
    R. finger flexion
    R. opponensplasty
    R. pollicization

Rippstein
    R. II technique

Ris·ser
    R. grade
    R. localizer
    R. sign

RL
    radiolunate (angle)

RLL
    radiolucent line
    right lower limb

R&M
    routine and microscopic

RMC un·con·strained de·vice

Rob·ert
    R's ligament
    R's pelvis

Rob·ert Brig·ham
    R.B. semiconstrained de-
      vice

Robert Jones
    R.J. bandage

Rob·erts
    Lloyd-R. osteotomy
    Lloyd-R. procedure
    R.-SC phocomelia syn-
      drome

Rob·ert·son
    Neal-R. litter

Ro·bi·ge·sic

Ro·bi·now
    R's syndrome

Rob·in·son
    R. catheter
    R. and Riley spinal fusion
    R. and Southwick cervical
        spinal fusion

Ro·bi·tet

Ro·ceph·in

rod
    Harrington r.
    Hunter r.
    interlocking r.
    intramedullary r.
    Knodt distraction r.
    Küntscher r.
    medullary r.
    muscle r.
    ratcheted r.
    Reverse Ratchet r.
    Rush r.
    Sage r.
    Schneider r.
    Universal r's
    Wissinger r.

Ro·di·chok
    R.'s classification

roent·gen

roent·geno·gram

roent·geno·graph

roent·geno·graph·ic

roent·gen·ol·o·gist

Rog·er
    R. cervical spinal fusion
    R's fusion

Rog·er An·der·son
    R.A. fixation device
    R.A. splint

Ro·ki·tan·sky
    R's pelvis
    R. sequence

Ro·lan·do
    R. fracture

roll
    axillary r.
    cotton r.
    plaster r.
    saggital r.

rollback
    femoral r.

Rol·lett
    R's secondary substance

ROM
    range of motion

Rom·berg
    R. test

Rome cri·te·ria

ROM ex·er·cis·es

ron·geur
    angled r.
    Beyer r.
    cervical r.
    Colclough laminectomy r.
    curved r.
    disk r.
    double-action r.
    Ferris-Smith r.
    Hodgson r.
    Kerrison r.
    laminectomy r.
    Leksell r.
    pituitary r.
    Schlesinger cervical r.
    single-action r.
    Spurling r.
    Stille r.
    Stille-Luer r.
    straight r.
    Takahashi r.

Roose·velt
    R. technique

root
    r. of arch of vertebra
    spinal nerve r.

Ro·per
R.-Tuke elbow prosthesis

Ro-Pro·fen

ro·sa·ry
rachitic r.

Rose
R. procedure
R.-Waaler test

Ro·sen
R. knife

Ro·sen·berg
Hench-R. syndrome

Ro·si·a·nu
Veleanu, R., and Ionescu
procedure

ro·ta·tion
external r.
instantaneous axis of r.
internal r.
saggital r. of vertebral
body
van Ness r.

Roth·man In·sti·tute to·tal
hip pros·the·sis

Roth·mund
R.-Thomson syndrome

Rou·bac

round·ing
r. of cranial border of vertebra

Roun·ox

Roux
R.-Goldthwait procedure

Rowe
Carter-R. view
Cave and R. procedure
Zarins and R. procedure

Roy
R.-Camille plate

Roy·flex

Royle
R.-Thompson thumb ad-
duction

RSA
roentgen stereophotogram-
metric analysis

RSD
reflex sympathetic dystrophy

R-T (Russell-Taylor)
reconstruction nail

Ru·bin·stein
R.-Taybi syndrome

Ru·da
Majestro, R., and Frost
procedure

ru·di·men·ta·ry

Ru·fen

Ru·iz
R.-Moro procedure

rul·er
Berndt hip r.

rup·ture
disk r.
foraminal disk r.
lateral disk r.
ligament r.

Rush
R. awl reamer
R. bender
R. driver-bender-extractor
R. pin
R. rod

Russe
Matti-R. graft
R. graft

Rus·sell
R. traction
R.-Silver syndrome

Rus·sell *(continued)*
    R.-Taylor interlocking nail
        system
    R.-Taylor nail

Rust
    R's disease
    R's phenomenon
    R's sign
    R's syndrome

Ru·val·ca·ba
    R. syndrome

Ru·val·ca·ba *(continued)*
    R.-Myhre syndrome

RVA
    rib vertebral angle

RVAD
    rib vertebral angle differ-
        ence

Ry·dell
    R. nail

Ry·er·son
    R. graft

S

S
    sacral vertebrae (S1–S5)

SAC
    short-arm cast

sac
    bursal s.
    dural s.
    thecal s.

SACH (solid-ankle cushioned
    heel) foot

Sachs
    Hill-S. fracture
    Hill-S. lesion
    S. nerve separator

sa·cral·gia

sa·cral·iza·tion

sa·crar·thro·gen·ic

sa·crec·to·my

sa·cro·coc·cy·ge·al

sa·cro·coc·cyx

sa·cro·cox·al·gia

sa·cro·cox·itis

sa·cro·dyn·ia

sa·cro·il·i·ac

sa·cro·il·i·itis

sa·cro·lis·the·sis

sa·cro·lum·bar

sa·cro·prom·on·to·ry

sa·cro·sci·at·ic

sa·cro·spi·nal

sa·crot·o·my

sa·cro·ver·te·bral

sa·crum
    assimilation s.
    tilted s.

Sad·don
    Brooks and S. procedure

Sae·thre
    S.-Chotzen syndrome

SAFE (stationary attachment
    flexible endoskeletal) foot

Sage
    S. rod

Sa·ger
    S. traction splint

Sa·ha
    S. procedure

St. George
    St. G. fully constrained de-
        vice
    St. G. sledge knee arthro-
        plasty
    St. G. sledge unicompart-
        mental device
    St. G.-Buchholz ankle
        prosthesis

Sal·a·zo·py·rin

Sal·flex

Sal·ge·sic

sal·i·cyl·ate

Sal·mo·nel·la

sal·sa·late

Sal·si·tab

salt
    bone s's

Sal·ter
    S. fracture
    S. osteotomy

Sal·ter *(continued)*
    S. sling
    S.-Harris classification
    S.-Harris fracture

Sal·ti·el
    S. orthosis

Salt·zer
    S. resurfacing procedure

sal·vage
    acetabular s.
    limb s.

Sal·va·ti
    Insall-S. ratio

San·fi·lip·po
    S's syndrome

san·gui·nous

sa·pon·i·fi·ca·tion

Sar·bó
    S. sign

sar·co·gen·ic

sar·coid
    Boeck's s.

sar·co·lem·ma

sar·co·lem·mic

sar·co·lem·mous

sar·co·ma *pl.* sar·co·mas, sar·co·ma·ta
    clear cell s.
    epithelioid s.
    Ewing's s.
    granulocytic s.
    osteoblastic s.
    osteogenic s.
    osteoid s.
    osteolytic s.
    pagetic s.
    parosteal s.
    periosteal s.
    reticulum cell s.
    synovial s.
    synovial cell s.

sar·co·mere

sar·co·plasm

sar·co·plas·mic

sar·co·plast

sar·co·poi·et·ic

sar·co·style

sar·co·tu·bules

sar·cous

Sar·gent
    S. procedure

Sar·mi·en·to
    S. osteotomy
    S. procedure
    S. total hip replacement

sar·to·ri·us

SAS
    short-arm splint

S.A.S.-500

S.A.S. En·ter·ic

Sat·ter·lee
    S. bone saw

sau·cer·iza·tion

saw
    Adams' s.
    amputating s.
    Butcher's s.
    cast s.
    end-cutting s.
    Gigli s.
    Hey's s.
    Luck-Bishop bone s.
    micro-oscillating s.
    oscillating s.
    reciprocating s.
    Satterlee bone s.
    Shrady's s.
    subcutaneous s.
    tangential s.

Sbar·baro
  S. tibial plateau prosthesis

SBO
  spina bifida occulta

scaf·fold

Sca·gli·et·ti
  S. reduction

scale
  Ficat grading s.
  Lynholm knee-scoring s.
  Marcus grading s.
  Marshall knee-scoring s.

sca·lene

sca·le·nec·to·my

sca·le·not·o·my

sca·le·nus

scal·lop·ing

scan
  bone s.
  bone-marrow s.
  gallium s.
  indium s.
  indium leukocyte s.
  technetium s.

scano·gram

sca·nog·ra·phy

scaph·oid
  bipartite s.
  humpback s.

scaph·oid·itis
  tarsal s.

scapho·lu·nate

scapho·tra·pe·zi·al

scap·u·la *pl.* scap·u·lae
  alar s.
  s. alata
  elevated s.
  Graves' s.
  scaphoid s.

scap·u·la *(continued)*
  winged s.

scap·u·lal·gia

scap·u·lar

scap·u·lec·to·my

scap·u·lo·cla·vic·u·lar

scap·u·lo·dyn·ia

scap·u·lo·hu·mer·al

scap·u·lo·pexy

scap·u·lo·tho·rac·ic

Scar·bor·ough
  S. total hip replacement

Scar·pa
  S's shoe
  ligament of S.

scar·ring
  epidural s.

sce·lal·gia

Schaef·fer
  S. orthosis

Schä·fer
  dumbbells of S.

Schanz
  S's disease
  S. osteotomy
  S's syndrome

Scheck
  Menson and S. procedure

Sche·de
  S's operation
  S. osteotomy

Scheie
  S's syndrome
  Hurler-S. compound syndrome

Scheier
  Gschwend, S., and Bahler
  elbow prosthesis

Schell·mann
  Klemm-S. locking nail

Scheu·er·mann
  S's disease
  S's kyphosis

Schin·zel
  S.-Giedion syndrome

Schlat·ter
  Osgood-S. disease
  S's sprain

Schlein
  S. elbow prosthesis

Schlemm
  S's ligaments

Schle·sin·ger
  S. cervical rongeur
  S. sign

Schmid
  metaphyseal chondrodys-
    plasia, S. type

Schmorl
  S. body
  S's disease
  S's node
  S's nodule

Schnei·der
  S. arthrodesis
  S. driver-extractor
  S. nail
  S. rod

Scho·ber
  S's index
  S's test

Schön·berg
  Albers-S. disease

school
  back s.

Schrei·ber
  S. maneuver

Schrock
  S. procedure

Schül·ler
  Hand-S.-Christian disease

Schul·tze
  S.-Chvostek sign

Schwann
  S. tumor

schwan·no·ma
  malignant s.
  spinal s.

Schwe·di·au·er
  S's disease

sci·at·ic

sci·at·i·ca

scin·ti·gram

scin·ti·graph

scin·ti·graph·ic

scin·tig·ra·phy
  bone s.

scis·sors
  cartilage s.
  Dean s.
  Mayo s.
  Metzenbaum s.
  suture s.

scle·ro·der·ma
  focal s.
  limited s.

scle·ro·des·mia

scle·ro·gen·ic

scle·rog·e·nous

scle·rose

scle·rosed

scle·ros·ing

scle·ro·sis
  amyotrophic lateral s.
  bone s.
  diaphyseal s.
  Mönckeberg's s.

scle·ro·sis *(continued)*
    multiple s.
    reactive s.

scle·ro·skel·e·ton

scle·ros·te·o·sis

scle·rot·ic

scle·ro·tom·al

scle·ro·tome

scle·ro·zone

SCOI shoul·der brace

sco·lio·ky·pho·sis

sco·lio·lor·do·sis

sco·lio·me·ter

sco·lio·ra·chit·ic

sco·lio·ra·chi·tis

sco·li·o·si·om·e·try

sco·li·o·sis
    acquired s.
    adolescent idiopathic s.
    Brissaud's s.
    cicatricial s.
    congenital s.
    coxitic s.
    degenerative s.
    empyematic s.
    fixed s.
    functional s.
    habit s.
    idiopathic s.
    infantile idiopathic s.
    inflammatory s.
    ischiatic s.
    juvenile idiopathic s.
    levorotary s.
    mobile s.
    myopathic s.
    ocular s.
    ophthalmic s.
    organic s.
    osteopathic s.
    paralytic s.

sco·li·o·sis *(continued)*
    rachitic s.
    rheumatic s.
    sciatic s.
    static s.
    uncompensated rotatory s.
    structural s.

sco·li·o·som·e·ter

sco·li·ot·ic

sco·lio·tone

sco·lop·sia

score
    Catterall hip s.
    Charnley s.
    Engh fixation s.
    Harris hip s.
    Lysholm knee s.
    Mayo hip s.

Scotch·cast

Scott
    S. procedure

Scot·tish Rite or·tho·sis

Sco·ville
    S. retractor

screw
    AO/ASIF lag s.
    cancellous s.
    compression s.
    compression hip s.
    compression lag s.
    cortical s.
    cruciate s.
    Eggers s.
    facet s.
    fixed-angle distraction s.
    Gore AO s.
    Henderson lag s.
    Herbert s.
    Herbert bone s.
    hex s.
    hip s.
    interference s.
    interfragmentary s.

screw *(continued)*
    Kurosaka s.
    lag s.
    Leinbach s.
    locking s.
    locking lag s.
    Lorenzo s.
    Martin s.
    McLaughlin s.
    patellar s.
    pedicle s.
    Phillips s.
    sacral s.
    Schanz s.
    set s.
    sliding s.
    spinal s.
    Steffee pedicle s.
    transfixion s.
    unicortical s.
    vertebral s.
    von Bahr s.
    Woodruff s.
    Zimmer compression hip s.

screw·driv·er
    angled s.
    automatic s.
    Flatt self-retaining s.
    Ken s.
    self-retaining s.

SCR (sin·gle com·part·ment)
re·place·ment knee

Scu·dari
    S. procedure

scu·tum
    s. pectoris

SD
    shoulder disarticulation

seam
    osteoid s.

Se·at·tle or·tho·sis

se·ba·ceous

se·cal·cif·er·ol

Seck·el
    S. syndrome

sec·tion·ing
    oblique s. of iliac crest

Sed·don
    S. arthrodesis

see·saw·ing

seg·ment
    motion s.
    posterior spinal muscle s.

seg·men·tal

seg·men·ta·tion
    unequal s.

seg·ment·ed

Se·gond
    S. fracture

seg·re·some

Sei·del
    S. nail

self-sus·pen·sion

Sel·ig
    S. procedure

SEM
    scanning electron micros-
    copy

semi·ca·nal
    s. of humerus

Semi-Cir·cu·lar gouge

semi·con·strained

semi·flex·ion

semi·lu·na·re

semi·lux·a·tion

semi·pen·ni·form

semi·ten·di·no·sus

Sen·e·gas
    S. approach

Senn
    S. double end retractor

Sen·sor·caine

Sen·ter
    S. syndrome

sep·a·ra·tion
    AC (acromioclavicular)
        joint s.
    fracture-s.
    joint s.
    shoulder s.
    traumatic chondral s.

sep·a·ra·tor
    nerve s.
    Sach's nerve s.

sep·sis

sep·tic

Sep·tra

sep·tum *pl.* sep·ta
    Bigelow's s.
    s. of Cloquet
    crural s.
    femoral s.
    s. femorale
    s. femorale [Cloqueti]
    intermuscular s., crural,
        anterior
    intermuscular s., crural,
        posterior
    intermuscular s. of arm,
        external
    intermuscular s. of arm,
        internal
    intermuscular s. of arm,
        lateral
    intermuscular s. of arm,
        medial
    intermuscular s. of leg,
        anterior
    intermuscular s. of leg,
        posterior
    intermuscular s. of thigh,
        external
    intermuscular s. of thigh,
        lateral

sep·tum *(continued)*
    intermuscular s. of thigh,
        medial
    s. intermusculare anterius
        cruris
    s. intermusculare brachii
        laterale
    s. intermusculare brachii
        mediale
    s. intermusculare cruris
        anterius
    s. intermusculare cruris
        posterius
    s. intermusculare femoris
        laterale
    s. intermusculare femoris
        mediale
    s. intermusculare humeri
        laterale
    s. intermusculare humeri
        mediale
    s. intermusculare poster-
        ius cruris

se·que·la *pl.* se·que·lae
    postpolio sequelae
    postpoliomyelitis sequelae

se·quence
    amyoplasia congenita s.
    amyoplasia congenita dis-
        ruptive s.
    Carpenter s.
    caudal dysplasia s.
    iniencephaly s.
    Klippel-Feil s.
    meningomyelocele s.
    moebius s.
    occult spinal dysraphism s.
    oligohydramnios s.
    Rotikansky s.
    sirenomelia s.

se·ques·ter

se·ques·tra

se·ques·tral

se·ques·tra·tion
    s. of disk

se·ques·trec·to·my

se·ques·trot·o·my

se·ques·trum *pl.* se·ques·tra
 primary s.
 secondary s.
 tertiary s.

se·ries
 lumbosacral s.
 Valpar component work
  sample s.

se·ro·pu·ru·lent

se·ro·san·guin·e·ous

se·ro·syn·o·vi·tis

se·rous

ser·ra·tus
 s. anterior

se·rum *pl.* se·rums, se·ra
 articular s.

ser·vice
 physical therapy s.

ses·a·moid

set
 phalangeal s.

Set·te·gast
 S's projection

set·tling
 cranial s.
 vertical s.

Se·ver
 Fairbanks and S. proce-
  dure
 S's disease

Se·ves·ta·no
 S. unicompartmental de-
  vice

SEWHO
 shoulder-elbow-wrist-hand
  orthosis

sex·dig·i·tate

SG
 serum globulin

SGP
 stress-generated potentials

Sh
 shoulder amputation

shaft
 s. of femur
 s. of fibula
 s. of humerus
 s. of metacarpal bone
 s. of metatarsal bone
 s. of phalanx of fingers
 s. of phalanx of toes
 s. of radius
 s. of rib
 s. of tibia
 s. of ulna

Shands
 MacEwen and S. osteot-
  omy

shank
 extended steel s.
 steel s.

Shanz
 S. dressing

shape
 Wiberg patellar s.

Sharp
 S.-Purser test

Shar·pey
 S's fibers

Shar·rard
 S. iliopsoas transfer
 S.-Trentani resurfacing
  procedure

shav·er
 arthroscopic s.
 bullet-nosed s.
 serrated suction s.

shav·ing
 femoral condylar s.

shav·ing *(continued)*
    patellar s.
    suction s.

shear

shears
    Bethune rib s.
    Gluck rib s.
    Liston s.
    rib s.
    Sauerbruch rib s.
    Shoemaker rib s.
    Stille-Giertz rib s.

sheath
    common s. of tendons of
      peroneal muscles
    fibrous s's of fingers
    fibrous s. of tendon
    fibrous s's of toes
    mucous s's
    mucous s., intertubercular
    mucous s. of tendon
    mucous s's of tendons of
      fingers
    mucous s's of tendons of
      toes
    s. of plantar tendon of long
      peroneal muscle
    synovial s. of bicipital
      groove
    synovial s. of intertubercu-
      lar groove
    synovial s. of tendon
    synovial s. of tendons of
      foot
    tendinous s's of flexor
      muscles of fingers
    tendinous s's of flexor
      muscles of toes
    tendinous s. of leg
    tendinous s. of long pero-
      neal muscle, plantar
    tendon s. of anterior tibial
      muscle
    tendon s's of long extensor
      muscles of toes

sheath *(continued)*
    tendon s's of long flexor
      muscles of toes
    tendon s. of posterior tibial
      muscle

Shee·han
    S. fully constrained device

sheet wad·ding

Shel·don
    Freeman-S. syndrome

shelf
    medial patellar s.

shell
    half s.
    internal eccentric s's

Shen·ton
    S. line

Shep·herd
    S's crook deformity
    S's fracture

Sher·man
    S. plate

shield
    amputation s.

shield·ing
    stress s.

Shiers
    S. fully constrained device

Shif·rin
    S. wire twister

shift
    central web skin volar
      dorsal s.
    Neer capsular s.
    pivot s.
    reverse pivot s.
    web space plasty s.

shim

shin
    cucumber s.

shin *(continued)*
    saber s.
    s. splints

shock
    spinal s.

shoe
    equinovarus outflare s.
    normal last s.
    reverse last s.
    Scarpa's s.
    space s.
    straight last s.
    wooden s.

Sho·keir
    Pena-S. phenotype

shoul·der
    s. apprehension
    apprehension s.
    Dana total s.
    disarticulation of s.
    dislocation of s.
    drop s.
    s. fracture
    frozen s.
    knocked-down s.
    Little Leaguer's s.
    loose s.
    Michael Reese Total S.
    Milwaukee s.
    s. orthosis
    ring man s.
    s. sprain
    stubbed s.
    s. subluxation

shoul·der-blade

show·er
    uric acid s.

Shprin·tzen
    S's syndrome

shrink·er
    stump s.

Sib·son
    S's aponeurosis

Sib·son *(continued)*
    S's fascia
    S's groove

side·port

Sif·fert
    S.-Foster-Nachamie proce-
        dure

sign
    Allis' s.
    Amoss' s.
    Achilles bulge s.
    Anghelescu's s.
    antecedent s.
    anterior apprehension s.
    anterior drawer s.
    anterior hiatal s.
    anterior tibial s.
    Ashhurst s.
    Babinski's s's
    bayonet s.
    Beevor's s.
    bowstring s.
    Bragard's s.
    Brudzinski's s.
    Bryant's s.
    Burton's s.
    camelback s.
    Chaddock's s.
    choppy sea s.
    Chvostek's s.
    Chvostek-Weiss s.
    Cleeman's s.
    Codman's s.
    cogwheel s.
    commemorative s.
    Comolli's s.
    contralateral s.
    Coopernail s.
    crescent s.
    Dawbarn's s.
    Dejerine's s.
    Demianoff's s.
    Desault's s.
    dimple s.
    doll's eye s.
    double camelback s.

sign *(continued)*
    drawer s.
    Dupuytren's s.
    Ely's s.
    Erichsen's s.
    external malleolar s.
    external malleolus s.
    fabere s.
    fadir s.
    Fajersztajn's crossed
      sciatic s.
    fan s.
    Finkelstein s.
    Fränkel's s.
    Froment's paper s.
    Gaenslen's s.
    Galeazzi s.
    Goldthwait's s.
    Gowers' s.
    Guilland's s.
    Hawkins s.
    Heberden's s's
    heel-cord s.
    Helbing's s.
    hiatal s.
    Hirschberg's s.
    Hoffmann's s.
    Homans' s.
    Hueter's s.
    Huntington's s.
    Kanavel's s.
    Keen's s.
    Kernig's s.
    Kerr's s.
    Langoria's s.
    Lasègue's s.
    Laugier's s.
    Leri's s.
    Lhermitte's s.
    Lichtenstern s.
    Linder's s.
    long tract s's
    Lorenz s.
    Ludloff's s.
    McMurray s.
    Maisonneuve's s.
    Marie-Foix s.
    Mennell's s.

sign *(continued)*
    Minor's s.
    Morquio's s.
    movie s.
    Murphy's s.
    Naffziger s.
    neck s.
    Nelson s.
    neurotension s.
    objective s.
    Oppenheim's s.
    Ortolani's s.
    Payr s.
    Phalen's s.
    physical s.
    piano key s.
    Piotrowski's s.
    piston s.
    posterior hiatal s.
    pronation s.
    pseudo-Babinski's s.
    Queckenstedt's s.
    radialis s.
    Raimiste's s.
    Risser s.
    Romberg's s.
    Rust's s.
    Sarbó's s.
    Schlesinger's s.
    Schultze-Chvostek s.
    signet ring s.
    somatic s.
    Soto-Hall s.
    spine s.
    stairs s.
    Strümpell's s.
    Strunsky's s.
    tension s.
    Thomas' s.
    tibialis s.
    Tinel's s.
    toe s.
    toe spread s.
    Trendelenburg's s.
    trough s.
    Turyn's s.
    Vanzetti's s.
    vital s's

sign *(continued)*
    Wartenberg's s.
    Weiss' s.
    windshield wiper s.

Si·las·tic

Si·le·si·an ban·dage

Si·le·si·an belt

Silfverskiöld
    S. procedure
    S's syndrome
    S. test

sil·i·cone
    s. elastomer
    HP-100 s. elastomer

Sil·ver
    Russell-S. syndrome
    S. operation
    S. procedure
    S.-Russell syndrome

Sim·mer·lin
    S's dystrophy
    S. type

Sim·mons
    S. test

Simms
    S.-Weinstein monofilament

Simp·son
    S. catheter

Sind·ing
    S.-Larsen-Johansson dis-
    ease

sin·ew
    weeping s.

Singh
    S. index

sin·is·ter

si·no·gram

si·nus *pl.* si·nus, si·nus·es
    articular s. of atlas

si·nus *(continued)*
    articular s. of atlas, supe-
    rior
    articular s. of axis, ante-
    rior
    articular s. of vertebrae,
    inferior
    s. of atlas, anterior
    s. condylorum femoris
    costal s's of sternum
    lunate s. of radius
    lunate s. of ulna
    middle s. of atlas
    peroneal s. of tibia
    semilunar s. of tibia
    tarsal s.
    s. tarsi

SIO
    sacroiliac orthosis

Sir·is
    Coffin-S. syndrome

Sisk
    Boyd and S. procedure

site
    donor s.

Si·vash
    S. total hip replacement

Si·we
    Letterer-S. disease

siz·er
    socket s.

Sjö·gren
    Marinesco-S. syndrome

ske·lal·gia

ske·las·the·nia

skel·e·ton
    appendicular s.
    s. appendiculare
    axial s.
    s. axiale
    s. membri inferioris liberi
    s. membri superioris liberi

skel·e·ton *(continued)*
    thoracic s.
    s. of thorax
    visceral s.

skew·foot

skid
    bone s.
    Murphy Lane bone s.

skill
    sensorimotor s.

Skil·lern
    S's fracture

SKI un·con·strained de·vice

skiv·ing

skull
    hot cross bun s.

SLAC
    scapholunate advanced
      collapse

SLAC wrist

SLAP (superior labrum
  anterior to posterior) le·sion

SLC
    short-leg cast

sleeve
    bridging s.
    excursion amplifier s.
    nerve s.
    polyethelene s.
    proximal s.
    rod s.

sling
    Glisson's s.
    pelvic s.
    Salter s.

slip
    tendon s.
    vertebral s.

slip·knot

Slo·cum
    S. procedure
    S. test

SLR
    straight leg raising

SLR test

SLS
    short-leg splint

SLWC
    short-leg walking cast

Sm-C
    somatomedin C

Smil·lie
    S. cartilage chisel
    S. cartilage knife
    S. nail
    S. retractor

Smith
    Ferris-S. rongeur
    Lyman-S. traction
    S. ankle prosthesis
    S's dislocation
    S's fracture
    S. physical capacities eval-
      uation
    S. total ankle replacement
    S.-Lemli-Opitz syndrome

Smith PCE
    Smith physical capacities
      evaluation

Smith-Pe·ter·sen
    S.-P. approach
    S.-P. arthrodesis
    S.-P. arthroplasty
    S.-P. gouge
    S.-P. nail
    S.-P. osteotome

Snook
    Chrisman and S. proce-
      dure

Snow
    S.-Litler procedure

snuff
    anatomical s.-box

SO
    shoulder orthosis

sock
    cast s.
    stump s.

sock·et
    check s.
    s. sizer
    suction s.

so·di·um
    s. fluoride
    gold s. thiomalate
    s. hydroxide
    s. phosphate P 32
    s. pyruvate
    s. salicylate
    s. urate

So·di·um Syn·flex

So·field
    S. osteotomy
    S. retractor

sole

so·le·us

Sol·ga·nal

so·lu·tion
    acid molybdate s.
    alkali s.
    aniline blue s.
    Biebrich scarlet–acid fuch-
        sin s.
    bis-tris buffer s.
    Bouin's s.
    hematoxylin s.
    hematoxylin s., Gill No. 3
    phosphorus standard s.
    sodium hydroxide s.
    sodium pyruvate s.
    Weigert's iron hematoxy-
        lin s.

so·ma·to·me·din

so·ma·to·tro·pin

Som·er·ville
    S. hip reduction

SOMI
    sternal-occipital-mandibu-
        lar immobilizer

SOMI or·tho·sis

so·no·gram

so·no·graph·ic

so·nog·ra·phy

sore
    pressure s.

Sor·ron·do
    S.-Ferré amputation

Soto-Hall
    S.-H. graft
    S.-H. sign
    West and S.-H. procedure

So·tos
    S. syndrome

Sou·ter
    S. elbow prosthesis

South·wick
    Robinson and S. cervical
        spinal fusion
    S. osteotomy
    S. slide procedure

Sout·ter
    S. procedure

space
    antecubital s.
    disk s.
    haversian s.
    intercostal s.
    interlaminar s.
    interosseous s's of meta-
        carpus
    interosseous s's of meta-
        tarsus
    marrow s.
    medullary s.

space *(continued)*
    midpalmar s.
    palmar s.
    Parona's s.
    periaxial s.
    popliteal s.
    predental s.
    subungual s.
    thenar s.
    web s.

spac·er
    Pheasant s.
    PMMA (polymethyl meth-
        acrylate) s.
    Silastic s.
    titanium-polyethylene s.
    wrist s.

spac·er block

spar·ing
    sacral s.

spasm
    muscle s.
    paravertebral s.
    paravertebral muscle s.

spas·tic

spa·ti·um *pl.* spa·tia
    s. intercostale
    spatia interossea meta-
        carpi
    spatia interossea meta-
        tarsi

SPE
    serum protein electropho-
        resis

spec
    spectroscopy

SPECT
    single photon emission
        computed tomography

spec·tros·co·py
    magnetic resonance s.

spec·trum *pl.* spec·tra
    facio-auriculo-vertebral s.
    oromandibular-limb hypo-
        genesis s.

Speed
    S. osteotomy
    S. procedure
    S's test
    S. and Boyd procedure

Spen·cer
    Borden, S., and Herndon
        osteotomy

sp gr
    specific gravity

Sphero·cen·tric ful·ly con·
    strained de·vice

spi·ca
    1½ s.
    double hip s.
    hip s.
    shoulder s.
    single hip s.
    three-finger s.
    thumb s.
    toe s.

spi·na *pl.* spi·nae
    s. bifida
    s. bifida occulta
    s. iliaca anterior inferior
    s. iliaca anterior superior
    s. iliaca posterior inferior
    s. iliaca posterior superior
    s. intercondyloidea
    s. ischiadica
    s. ischialis
    s. scapulae
    s. tibiae

spi·nal

spi·nal·gia

spi·na·lis

Spi·nal-Stim

spine
    anterior tibial s.
    anterosuperior iliac s.
    bamboo s.
    cervical s.
    coccygeal s.
    deformed s.
    dorsal s.
    s. of greater tubercle of
      humerus
    iliopectineal s.
    intercondyloid s.
    ischial s.
    s. of ischium
    kissing s's
    s. of lesser tubercle of hu-
      merus
    lumbar s.
    neural s.
    obturator s.
    peroneal s. of os calcis
    poker s.
    posterior tibial s.
    s. of pubic bone
    s. of pubis
    rigid s.
    rugger jersey s.
    sacral s.
    s. of scapula
    sciatic s.
    thoracic s.
    s. of tibia
    tibial s.
    trochanteric s., greater
    trochanteric s., lesser
    typhoid s.
    s. of vertebra

Spi·nel·li
    Monticelli-S. fixation de-
      vice

Spi·nex

spi·no·cos·tal·is

spi·no·gle·noid

Spira
    S. procedure

Spitt·ler
    S. procedure
    S. and McFaddin amputa-
      tion

splay·foot

sple·ni·al

splen·i·ser·rate

splint
    adjustable Thomas s.
    air s.
    air pressure s.
    airplane s.
    aluminum foam s.
    Anderson s.
    Balkan s.
    banjo traction s.
    baseball s.
    Bennett basic hand s.
    Böhler s.
    Böhler-Braun s.
    Chandler felt collar s.
    coaptation s's
    cockup s.
    Cramer's s.
    Denis Browne s.
    drop foot s.
    dynamic s.
    Engen palmar basic
      wrist s.
    fist s.
    Frejka pillow s.
    frog s.
    functional s.
    gutter s.
    hairpin s.
    half-ring Thomas s.
    hayrake s.
    Hodgen s.
    Ilfeld s.
    inflatable s.
    Kanavel's cockup s.
    Keller-Blake s.
    Kenny-Howard s.
    Kirschner wire s.
    ladder s.
    Liston's s.

splint *(continued)*
    long-arm s.
    long-leg s.
    mallet-finger s.
    Morris external fixation s.
    night s.
    opponens s.
    pillow s.
    plaster s.
    plastic s.
    poroplastic s.
    posterior s.
    Pugifix fist s.
    Roger Anderson s.
    Sager traction s.
    shin s.
    shin s's
    short-arm s.
    short-leg s.
    Stader s.
    static s.
    sugar-tong s.
    talipes hobble s.
    Taylor s.
    Thomas s.
    Thomas knee s.
    Tobruk s.
    traction s.
    universal gutter s.
    Velcro s.
    volar s.
    von Rosen s.
    Warm Springs rachet
        flexor tenodesis s.
    wraparound s.

splin·ter

splint·ing

splints
    shin s.

spon·dy·lal·gia

spon·dyl·ar·thri·tis
    s. ankylopoietica

spon·dyl·ar·throc·a·ce

spon·dyl·ex·ar·thro·sis

spon·dy·lit·ic

spon·dy·li·tis
    s. ankylopoietica
    s. ankylosans
    ankylosing s.
    Bekhterev's s.
    s. deformans
    enteropathic s.
    hypertrophic s.
    s. infectiosa
    Kümmell's s.
    Marie-Strümpell s.
    muscular s.
    mycotic s.
    post-traumatic s.
    psoriatic s.
    pyogenic s.
    rheumatoid s.
    rhizomelic s.
    s. rhizomelica
    s. rhizomélique
    traumatic s.
    s. tuberculosa
    tuberculous s.
    s. typhosa

spon·dy·li·ze·ma

spon·dy·lo·ar·throp·a·thy

spon·dy·loc·a·ce

spon·dy·lo·dyn·ia

spon·dy·lo·gen·ic

spon·dy·lo·lis·the·sis
    congenital s.
    degenerative s.
    dysplastic s.
    isthmic s.
    lytic s.
    pathological s.
    traumatic s.

spon·dy·lo·lis·thet·ic

spon·dy·lol·y·sis

spon·dy·lo·ma·la·cia
    s. traumatica

spon·dy·lo·meg·a·ly

spon·dy·lop·a·thy
    traumatic s.

spon·dy·lop·to·sis

spon·dy·lo·py·o·sis

spon·dy·los·chi·sis

spon·dy·lo·sis
    cervical s.
    s. chronica ankylopoietica
    lumbar s.
    rhizomelic s.
    s. uncovertebralis

spon·dy·lo·syn·de·sis

spon·dy·lot·ic

spon·dy·lot·o·my
    Callahan s.

spon·dy·lous

spon·gio·sa

spon·gio·sa·plas·ty

spot
    café au lait s's

sprain
    ankle s.
    anterior cruciate s.
    deltoid s.
    knee s.
    lateral collateral s.
    medial collateral s.
    posterior cruciate s.
    posterior oblique s.
    rider's s.
    Schlatter's s.
    shoulder s.
    tibiofibular s.

spread·er
    Cloward intervertebral s.
    lamina s.
    laminar s.

Spren·gel
    S's deformity

spring
    Weiss s's

Spring·er
    S's fracture

spur
    bone s.
    bony s.
    calcaneal s.
    chondro-osseous s.
    heel s.
    occipital s.
    olecranon s.
    traction s.

Spur·ling
    S. rongeur
    S. test

spur·ring
    anterior s.

Spur·way
    S. syndrome

squat·ting

S-ROM fem·o·ral pros·the·sis

S-ROM Su·per·Cup

sta·bil·i·ty
    distal s.
    rotational s.
    viscoelastic s.

sta·bil·iza·tion
    cervical s.
    spinal s.

sta·bi·li·zer
    joint s.

Sta·bilo·con·dy·lar semi·con·
strained de·vice

Stack
    Magnuson-S. procedure

Sta·der
    S. splint

stag·ing
    TNM s.

Stag·nara
S. view

Sta·he·li
S. procedure

stain
CPK Agaro-S.
Gomori's s's
Gram's s.
Masson s.
trichrome s.

Stamm
S. arthrodesis

stance

Sta·nis·lav·je·vic
S. procedure

Stan·more
S. elbow prosthesis
S. fully constrained device
S. total hip replacement

Staph·y·lo·coc·cus
S. aureus

sta·ple
Blount s.
s. inserter

Sta·ples
S. arthrodesis
S.-Black-Brostrom procedure

stap·ling
epiphyseal s.

start·er
nail s.

Sta·tak
S. device

stat·ic

sta·tus
s. arthriticus

steel
stainless s.

Steel·quist
King and S. amputation

Stef·fe
S. arthroplasty
S. pedicle screw
S. plate

Stein
Gill-S. arthrodesis

Stein·brock·er
S's syndrome

Steind·ler
S. arthrodesis
S. flexorplasty
S. matricectomy
S. procedure

Stei·ner
S's tumors

Stein·ert
S. myotonic dystrophy
syndrome

Stein·mann
S. pin
S. pin holder
S. pin retractor
S. threaded pin

stem
femoral s.

Sten·er
S. and Gunterberg procedure

ste·no·sis
degenerative lumbar s.
lateral recess s.
spinal s.
spinal canal s.

stent

ster·eo·ar·throl·y·sis

Steri-strip

ster·nal

ster·nal·gia

Stern·berg
   Albright-McCune-S. syn-
      drome
   Reed-S. cells

ster·nen

ster·no·cla·vic·u·lar

ster·no·cla·vic·u·la·ris

ster·no·clei·dal

ster·no·clei·do·mas·toid

ster·no·clei·do·mas·toi·de·us

ster·no·cos·tal

ster·no·dyn·ia

ster·no·mas·toid

ster·no·scap·u·lar

ster·not·o·my

ster·no·try·pe·sis

ster·no·ver·te·bral

ster·num
   s. bifidum
   cleft s.

stetho·my·itis

stetho·my·o·si·tis

Ste·wart
   S. procedure
   S. and Harley arthrodesis
   S.-Morel syndrome

STH-2 to·tal hip re·place·
   ment

Stick·ler
   S. syndrome

Stie·da
   Pellegrini-S. disease
   S's disease
   S's fracture
   S's process

stiff·ness
   joint s.

stiff·ness *(continued)*
   morning s.

Stif·neck
   S. collar

stig·ma *pl.* stig·mas, stig·ma·
   ta

Stiles
   S.-Bunnell finger flexion

Still
   S's disease

Stille
   S. rongeur
   S.-Liston bone cutting for-
      ceps
   S.-Luer rongeur

Stil·ler
   S's rib

Stil·phos·trol

Stim·son
   S. maneuver

stim·u·la·tion
   electrical s. of fracture
      healing
   functional electrical s.
   functional neuro-
      muscular s.
   magnetic s. of fracture
      healing
   transcutaneous electrical
      nerve s. (TENS)

stim·u·la·tor
   AME bone growth s.
   bone growth s.

stir·rup
   split s.

stitch
   Bunnell s.

stitch·er
   Arthrex grasping s.
   grasping s.

stock·i·nette

Stokes
  S's amputation
  S. operation

Stoll
  S. test

Stone
  S. arthrodesis
  S. procedure

stone
  chalk s.

stop
  MP s.

stor·i·form

strain
  cervical s.
  muscle s.
  normal s.
  shear s.

strait
  pelvic s., inferior
  pelvic s., superior

strap
  buddy s.
  chest s.
  fork s.
  infrapatellar s.
  suprapatellar s.
  valgus corrective ankle s.
  varus corrective ankle s.

strap·ping
  Gibney's s.

stra·tum *pl.* stra·ta
  s. fibrosum capsulae arti-
    cularis
  s. fibrosum vaginae tendi-
    nis
  s. synoviale capsulae arti-
    cularis
  s. synoviale vaginae tendi-
    nis

Straub
  Thomas, Thompson, and S.
    procedure

Stray·er
  S. procedure
  S. technique

streb·lo·mi·cro·dac·ty·ly

Street
  Hansen-S. driver-extractor
  Hansen-S. nail
  S. medullary pin

Stree·ter
  S's dysplasia

Streiff
  Hallermann-S. syndrome

strength
  fatigue s.

streph·eno·po·dia

streph·exo·po·dia

strepho·po·dia

Strep·to·coc·cus

strep·to·mi·cro·dac·ty·ly

strep·to·my·cin
  s. hydrochloride
  s. sulfate

stress
  allowable s.
  bursting s.
  inversion ankle s.
  normal s.
  push-pull ankle s.
  shear s.
  torsional s.
  yield s.

stress-re·lax·a·tion

stria *pl.* striae
  striae of Amici

strike
  heel s.

strip·per
    tendon s.

struc·ture
    osseous s.

Strüm·pell
    Marie-S. disease
    Marie-S. spondylitis
    S's sign
    S.-Marie disease

Strun·sky
    S. sign

Struth·ers
    ligament of S.

Stry·ker frame

Stry·ker/OSI laxity tester

STS
    serologic test for syphilis

STSG
    split thickness skin graft

Stull·berg
    S. method

stump
    Boyd s.
    conical s.
    Pirogoff s.
    s. shrinker
    Syme s.

sty·loi·dec·to·my
    radial s.

sty·los·teo·phyte

sub·ac·e·tab·u·lar

sub·acro·mi·al

sub·apo·neu·rot·ic

sub·as·trag·a·lar

Sub·ba·Row
    Fiske and S. reducer

sub·cap·su·lo·peri·os·te·al

sub·chon·dral

sub·cor·a·coid

sub·cu·ta·ne·ous

sub·cu·tic·u·lar

sub·il·i·um

sub·lam·i·nar

sub·lim·i·nal

sub·lux

sub·lux·ate

sub·lux·a·tion
    atlantoaxial s.
    chronic s.
    facet s.
    occult s.
    s. of patella
    radioulnar s.
    rotary s.
    sacroiliac s.
    subaxial s.
    tendon s.
    translational s.
    unilateral facet s.
    Volkmann's s.
    wrist s.

sub·pa·tel·lar

sub·peri·os·te·al

sub·peri·os·teo·cap·su·lar

sub·phase
    loading response s.

sub·scap·u·lar·is

sub·spi·nous

sub·stance
    compact s. of bones
    cortical s. of bone
    medullary s. of bone
    medullary s. of bone, red
    medullary s. of bone, yel-
        low
    Rollett's secondary s.
    sarcous s.
    spongy s. of bone

sub·stance *(continued)*
    trabecular s. of bone

sub·stan·tia *pl.* sub·stan·tiae
    s. compacta ossium
    s. corticalis ossium
    s. spongiosa ossium
    s. trabecularis ossium

sub·sti·tute
    plasma s.

sub·sti·tu·tion
    creeping s.
    creeping s. of bone

sub·ta·lar

sub·tar·sal

sub·tro·chan·ter·ic

sub·un·gual

sub·unit
    proteoglycan s.

sub·ver·te·bral

su·cral·fate

Su·deck
    S. atrophy
    S's disease

sug·ar
    fasting blood s.

Su·gi·u·ka
    S. osteotomy

Sukh·tian
    S.-Hughes fixation device

Su·kul
    S. classification (for scaphoid nonunion)

Sul·crate

sul·cus *pl.* sul·ci
    s. arteriae subclaviae
    s. arteriae vertebralis atlantis
    bicipital s., lateral
    bicipital s., medial

sul·cus *(continued)*
    bicipital s., radial
    bicipital s., ulnar
    s. bicipitalis lateralis
    s. bicipitalis medialis
    s. bicipitalis radialis
    s. bicipitalis ulnaris
    calcaneal s.
    s. calcanei
    carpal s.
    s. carpi
    s. costae
    costal s.
    costal s., inferior
    cuboid s.
    femoral s.
    hypoplastic femoral s.
    interarticular s. of calcaneus
    interarticular s. of talus
    intertubercular s. of humerus
    s. intertubercularis humeri
    malleolar s. of fibula
    malleolar s. of tibia
    s. malleolaris fibulae
    s. malleolaris tibiae
    s. musculi flexoris hallucis longi calcanei
    s. musculi flexoris hallucis longi tali
    s. musculi peronaei calcanei
    s. musculi peronaei ossis cuboidei
    s. musculi subclavii
    s. nervi radialis
    s. nervi spinalis
    s. nervi ulnaris
    obturator s. of pubis
    s. obturatorius ossis pubis
    paraglenoid sulci of hip bone
    sulci paraglenoidales ossis coxae
    radial s. of humerus
    s. of radial nerve

sul·cus *(continued)*
    s. of semicanal of humerus
    semilunar s. of radius
    spiral s.
    spiral s. of humerus
    s. spiralis
    s. subclaviae
    subclavian s.
    s. of subclavian artery
    subclavian s. of lung
    s. for subclavian muscle
    s. of subclavian vein
    s. subclavius
    supra-acetabular s.
    s. supra-acetabularis
    s. tali
    s. of talus
    s. tendinis musculi flexoris
      hallucis longi calcanei
    s. tendinis musculi flexoris
      hallucis longi tali
    s. tendinis musculi peronei
      longi
    s. tendinum musculorum
      fibularium calcanei
    s. tendinum musculorum
      peroneorum calcanei
    s. of tendon of flexor hallu-
      cis longus muscle of cal-
      caneus
    s. of tendon of flexor hallu-
      cis longus muscle of talus
    s. of tendons of peroneus
      muscles
    s. of tendon of peroneus
      longus muscle
    s. of ulnar nerve
    s. venae subclaviae
    s. of vertebral artery of at-
      las
    s. of wrist

Sul·fa·meth·o·prim

sul·fa·meth·ox·a·zole
    s. and trimethoprim

Sul·fa·prim

sul·fa·sal·a·zine

sul·fate
    keratin s.

Sul·fa·trim

Sul·fox·a·prim

sul·in·dac

Su·my·cin

su·per·ab·duc·tion

su·per·acro·mi·al

su·per·al·loy

Su·per·Cup ac·e·tab·u·lar
    cup

su·per·ex·tend·ed

su·per·ex·ten·sion

su·per·fi·cial

su·per·flex·ion

su·per·gen·u·al

su·pe·ri·or

su·per·nu·mer·ary

su·pero·lat·er·al

su·pi·na·tion

su·pi·na·tion-ad·duc·tion

su·pi·na·tion-ever·sion

su·pi·na·tor

su·pine

Sup·pan
    S. procedure

sup·port
    arch s.
    Arizona universal leg s.
    combined arch s.
    double s.
    metatarsal s.
    plantar arch s.

sup·pu·ra·tive

su·pra-acro·mi·al

su·pra·con·dy·lar

su·pra·con·dy·loid

su·pra·cos·tal

su·pra·cot·y·loid

su·pra·epi·con·dy·lar

su·pra·epi·troch·le·ar

su·pra·gle·noid

su·pra·mal·le·o·lar

su·pra·pa·tel·lar

su·pra·scap·u·lar

su·pra·spi·na·tus

Su·prax

Sure·Tac de·vice

sur·face
   anterior s. of manubrium
     and gladiolus
   anterior s. of sacral bone
   anterior s. of scapula
   anterior talar articular s.
   articular s.
   articular s. of acetabulum
   articular s. of sacral bone,
     lateral
   auricular s. of sacrum
   carpal articular s.
   condyloid s. of tibia
   costal s.
   costal s. of scapula
   cuboid articular s.
   dorsal s.
   dorsal s. of scapula
   extensor s.
   flexor s.
   plantar s.
   posterior s. of sacral bone
   posterior s. of scapula
   sacropelvic s. of the ilium
   superior articular s. of at-
     las
   symphysial s.
   ventral s.

sur·face *(continued)*
   ventral s. of scapula
   volar s.

Sur·gam

sur·geon
   hand s.
   orthopaedic (orthopedic) s.

sur·gery
   cineplastic s.
   disk s.
   limb-salvage s.
   limb-sparing s.
   minimal intervention s.
   orthopaedic (orthopedic) s.
   vascular s.

Sur·gi·cel

sus·pen·sion
   above-knee s.
   balanced s.
   below-knee s.
   hemipelvectomy s.
   knee disarticulation s.
   overhead s.

sus·pen·sion·plas·ty

sus·ten·tac·u·lum *pl.* sus·
ten·tac·u·la
   s. tali
   s. of talus

Suth·er·land
   S. procedure
   S. tendon transfer
   S.-Greenfield osteotomy

su·tu·ra *pl.* su·tu·rae

su·ture
   absorbable s.
   Bunnell's s.
   chromic gut s.
   cotton s.
   Czerny's s.
   Dacron s.
   Dexon s.
   double-loop s.
   double-weave s.

su·ture *(continued)*
 Ethibond s.
 Kessler s.
 Krackow s.
 Le Dentu's s.
 Le Fort's s.
 Maxon s.
 nonabsorbable s.
 nylon s.
 s. passer
 PDS s.
 polydioxanone s.
 polyester s.
 polyester fiber s.
 polyethylene s.
 pullout s.
 s. retriever
 silk s.
 stainless steel s.
 Tycron s.
 Vicryl s.

Swan·son
 Freeman-S. unconstrained
  device
 S. arthroplasty
 S. carpal scaphoid implant
 S. implant
 S. prosthesis
 S. tendon passer
 S. toe joint

sway
 lateral s.

sway·back

Swe·dish knee cage

swell·ing
 blennorrhagic s.

Swis·chuk
 spinolaminar line of S.

Syme
 S's amputation
 S's operation
 S. stump

sym·met·ric

sym·pha·lan·gia

sym·pha·lan·gism
 multiple s.

sym·phys·e·al

sym·phys·e·or·rha·phy

sym·phy·ses

sym·phys·i·al

sym·phys·i·or·rha·phy

sym·phy·sis *pl.* sym·phy·ses
 intervertebral s.
 s. intervertebralis
 manubriosternal s.
 s. manubriosternalis
 s. ossium pubis
 pubic s.
 s. pubica
 s. pubis
 s. sacrococcygea
 sacrococcygeal s.
 sacroiliac s.

symp·tom
 low back s's
 Trendelenburg's s.

syn·ar·thro·dia

syn·ar·thro·di·al

syn·ar·thro·phy·sis

syn·ar·thro·ses

syn·ar·thro·sis *pl.* syn·ar·
 thro·ses

syn·chon·dro·sis *pl.* syn·
 chon·dro·ses
 costoclavicular s.
 manubriosternal s.
 s. manubriosternalis
 pubic s.
 s. pubis
 sacrococcygeal s.
 sternal s.
 s. sternalis

syn·chon·drot·o·my

syn•co•pe

syn•dac•ty•li•za•tion

syn•dac•ty•ly
    complex s.
    first web space s.
    simple s.

syn•de•sis

syn•des•mec•to•my
    s. metatarsea

syn•des•mo-odon•toid

syn•des•mo•pexy

syn•des•mo•phyte

syn•des•mo•plas•ty

syn•des•mor•rha•phy

syn•des•mo•sis *pl.* syn•des•
  mo•ses
    radioulnar s.
    s. radio-ulnaris
    tibiofibular s.
    s. tibiofibularis

syn•des•mot•o•my

syn•drome (see also under
  disease)
    Aarskog s.
    Aase s.
    achondrogenesis s's
    Adams-Oliver s.
    Albright's s.
    Albright-McCune-Stern-
      berg s.
    amniotic band s.
    anterior compartment s.
    anterior cord s.
    anterior fat pad s.
    anterior interosseous s.
    Antley-Bixler s.
    Apert's s.
    Arnold-Chiari s.
    Baastrup's s.
    Babinski-Fröhlich s.
    Baller-Gerold s.
    Bardet-Biedl s.

syn•drome *(continued)*
    Beals' s.
    Beals' auriculo-osteodys-
      plasia s.
    Behçet's s.
    Bertolotti's s.
    black heel s.
    Bloom s.
    blue toe s.
    Börjeson-Forssman-Leh-
      mann s.
    brachydactyly s.
    brachydactyly s., type E
    brittle bone s.
    Brown-Séquard s.
    camptomelic s.
    Camurati-Englemann s.
    carpal tunnel s.
    Carpenter's s.
    cast s.
    cat-eye s.
    cat's eye s.
    cauda equina s.
    central cord s.
    cerebrocostomandibular s.
    cerebro-oculo-facio-
      skeletal s.
    CHILD s.
    Cockayne's s.
    Coffin-Lowry s.
    Coffin-Siris s.
    Cohen's s.
    compartment s.
    Conradi's s.
    Conradi-Hünermann s.
    cord impingement s's
    costoclavicular s.
    craniomandibular
      cervical s.
    CREST s.
    Crouzon s.
    cubital tunnel s.
    Cyriax's s.
    dead arm s.
    de Lange's s.
    de Quervain s.
    disk s.
    disk disruption s.

syn·drome *(continued)*
  distal arthrogryposis s.
  double-crush s.
  Down s.
  Dubowitz s.
  Dyggve-Melchior-
    Clausen s.
  dyskeratosis congenita s.
  EEC s.
  Ehlers-Danlos s.
  entrapment s.
  Escobar s.
  excessive lateral
    pressure s.
  facet s.
  Fanconi's s.
  Fanconi's pancytopenia s.
  Felty's s.
  femoral hypopla-
    sia—unusual facies s.
  FG s.
  fibrodysplasia ossificans
    progressiva s.
  flexor origin s.
  fragile X s.
  Fraser s.
  Freeman-Sheldon s.
  Gardner's s.
  generalized gangliosidosis
    s., type I
  Goltz s.
  Gorlin's s.
  Grebe s.
  Greig cephalopolysyndac-
    tyly s.
  Guillain-Barré s.
  Hajdu-Cheney s.
  Hallermann-Streiff s.
  Hay-Wells s.
  Hecht s.
  Hench-Rosenberg s.
  Holt-Oram s.
  homocystinuria s.
  Hunter's s.
  Hurler s.
  Hurler-Scheie compound s.
  hyperlaxity s.
  impingement s.

syn·drome *(continued)*
  incontinentia pigmenti s.
  intramedullary s.
  Jaccoud's s.
  Jaffe-Lichtenstein s.
  Jarcho-Levin s.
  Kast's s.
  Killian and Teschler-Ni-
    cola s.
  Klinefelter's s.
  Klippel-Feil s.
  Klippel-Trenaunay-
    Weber s.
  Langer-Giedion s.
  Larsen's s.
  lateral facet s.
  lateral recess s.
  Legg-Calvé-Perthes s.
  Lenz-Majewski s.
  Lenz-Majewski hyperosto-
    sis s.
  Leroy I-cell s.
  lethal multiple
    pterygium s.
  Levy-Hollister s.
  Leyden-Moebius s.
  Lobstein's s.
  Looser-Milkman s.
  Lowe s.
  lumbar thecoperitoneal
    shunt s.
  lupus-like s.
  McCune-Albright s.
  Maffucci's s.
  malalignment s.
  Marfan s.
  Marie s.
  Marie-Bamberger s.
  Marinesco-Sjögren's s.
  Maroteaux-Lamy s.
  Maroteaux-Lamy muco-
    polysaccharidosis s.
  Marshall's s.
  Meckel-Gruber s.
  medial shelf s.
  Melnick-Needles s.
  Menkes' s.
  Mietens s.

syn·drome *(continued)*
- milk-alkali s.
- Milkman's s.
- Miller s.
- Miller-Dieker s.
- Mohr s.
- Morel's s.
- Morquio s.
- Morton's s.
- multiple exostoses s.
- multiple lentigines s.
- multiple neuroma s.
- multiple synostosis s.
- Naffziger's s.
- Nager s.
- nail-patella s.
- neurofibromatosis s.
- Noonan's s.
- oculodentodigital s.
- oligohydramnios s.
- oral-facial-digital s.
- oropalatodigital s.
- osteochondromatosis s.
- osteogenesis imperfecta s., type I
- osteogenesis imperfecta s., type II
- Ostrum-Furst s.
- otopalatodigital s., type I
- otopalatodigital s., type II
- overuse s.
- 4p⁻ s.
- 5p⁻ s.
- 9p⁻ s.
- 18p⁻ s.
- painful arc s.
- Pancoast's s.
- Pallister-Hall s.
- Parsonage-Turner s.
- partial trisomy 10q s.
- patellar clunk s.
- patellar pain s.
- patellofemoral s.
- Pellegrini-Stieda s.
- Pfeiffer's s.
- plica s.
- Poland's s.
- popliteal pterygium s.

syn·drome *(continued)*
- popliteal web s.
- postphlebitic s.
- postphlebitis s.
- Prader-Willi s.
- progeria s.
- pronator s.
- Proteus s.
- pseudo-Felty's s.
- pseudo-Hurler polydystrophy s.
- pyriformis s.
- 12q⁻ s.
- 13q⁻ s.
- 18q⁻ s.
- radial aplasia–thrombocytopenia s.
- radicular s.
- rectus femoris s.
- Reiter's s.
- rhizomelic chondrodysplasia punctata s.
- Riley-Day s.
- Roberts-SC phocomelia s.
- Robinow's s.
- Rothmund-Thomson s.
- Rubinstein-Taybi s.
- Russell-Silver s.
- Rust's s.
- Ruvalcaba's s.
- Saethre-Chotzen s.
- Sanfilippo's s.
- scapulocostal s.
- Schanz's s.
- Scheie's s.
- Schinzel-Giedion s.
- Schwartz-Jampel s.
- Seckel's s.
- Senter s.
- shoulder-hand s.
- Shprintzen's s.
- Silfverskiöld's s.
- SLE-like s.
- Smith-Lemli-Opitz s.
- Sotos' s.
- Spurway s.
- Steinbrocker's s.

syn·drome *(continued)*
    Steinert myotonic dystro-
      phy s.
    Stewart-Morel s.
    Stickler s.
    stiff-man s.
    straight back s.
    Sudeck-Leriche s.
    superior mesenteric
      artery s.
    supraspinatus s.
    TAR (thrombocytope-
      nia–absent radius) s.
    temporomandibular
      joint s.
    Thiele s.
    Thiemann's s.
    thoracic outlet s.
    Tietze's s.
    TMJ (temporomandibular
      joint) s.
    Touraine-Solente-Golé s.
    Townes' s.
    trichorhinophalangeal s.
    triploidy s.
    trisomy 4p s.
    trisomy 8 s.
    trisomy 9 mosaic s.
    trisomy 9p s.
    trisomy 13 s.
    trisomy 18 s.
    trisomy 20p s.
    Turner's s.
    van Buchem's s.
    Volkmann's s.
    Waardenburg's s.
    Weaver s.
    Weill-Marchesani s.
    Werner s.
    Williams s.
    X-linked hydrocephalus s.
    XO s.
    XXXX s.
    XXXXX s.
    XXXXY s.
    XXY s.
    XYY s.
    Zellweger s.

syn·neu·ro·sis

syn·os·te·ol·o·gy

syn·os·te·o·sis

syn·os·te·ot·ic

syn·os·te·ot·o·my

syn·os·to·sis *pl.* syn·os·to·ses
    radioulnar s.
    tarsal s.

syn·os·tot·ic

syn·o·vec·to·my
    posterior s.

sy·no·via

sy·no·vi·al

sy·no·vi·a·lis

sy·no·vin

sy·no·vio·blast

sy·no·vio·chon·dro·ma·to·sis

sy·no·vio·cyte

sy·no·vi·o·ma

syn·o·vip·a·rous

syno·vi·tis
    bursal s.
    dendritic s.
    dry s.
    fungous s.
    granulomatous s.
    intramedullary s.
    localized nodular s.
    pigmented villonodular s.
    purulent s.
    serous s.
    s. sicca
    silicone s.
    simple s.
    tendinous s.
    vaginal s.
    vibration s.
    villonodular s.
    villous s.

sy·no·vi·um
  rheumatoid s.

syn·phal·an·gism

syn·tax·is

syn·te·no·sis

syn·the·sis
  collagen s.

syn·trip·sis

sy·rin·go·my·e·lia

sys·tem
  Acufex screw s.
  C-D (Cotrel-Dubousset) s.
  capsuloligamentous s.
  central nervous s. (CNS)
  cerebrospinal s.
  d'Aubigne scoring s.
  Edwards Modular
    Spinal S.
  endoskeletal prosthetic s.
  Evolution Total Hip S.
  Exact-Fit ATH s.
  haversian s.
  Hex-Fix external
    fixation s.
  Hydroxylapatite Mc-
    Cutchen Total Hip S.
  Insall/Burstein II modular
    knee s.
  Integral hip replace-
    ment s.
  Integrated Shape
    Imaging S.

sys·tem *(continued)*
  intermediate prosthetic s.
  interstitial s.
  ISOLA Spinal S.
  Kinemax Plus Total
    Knee S.
  Kostuik-Harrington s.
  McCutchen SLT Total
    Hip S.
  modular prosthetic s.
  muscular s.
  musculoskeletal s.
  musculotendinous s.
  nervous s.
  neuromuscular s.
  Nexus Total Hip S.
  Partridge cerclene s.
  peripheral nervous s.
  PFC Total Hip S.
  Poly-Dial insert s.
  Pro-Trac cruciate recon-
    struction s.
  Russell-Taylor interlock-
    ing nail s.
  skeletal s.
  T s.
  temporary prosthetic s.
  Transtibial drill guide s.
  triad s.
  vascular s.
  ZMS intramedullary fixa-
    tion s.

sys·te·ma
  s. skeletale

sys·to·le

sys·trem·ma

T
thoracic vertebrae
(T1–T12)
thorax

T₃
triiodothyronine

T₄
thyroxine

Ta
tarsus
tarsal amputation

TAA
total ankle arthroplasty

ta·ba·tière ana·to·mique

Ta·ber
Carroll and T. arthro-
plasty

ta·bes
t. dorsalis

ta·ble
fracture t.
hand t.
resistive exercise t.
spinal surgery t.

ta·bo·pa·ral·y·sis

ta·bo·pa·re·sis

Tach·djian
T. orthosis
T. tendon transfer

tack
absorbable t.
cannulated t.

Taft
Pulver-T. finger flexion

tail
occult t.

Tait
T. flap
T. graft

Ta·ka·ha·shi
T. rongeur

Ta·ka·hu·ra
T. total ankle replacement

TAL
tendo Achillis lengthening

tal·al·gia

ta·lar

tal·ec·to·my
Whitman t.

ta·li

tal·i·ped

tal·i·pe·dic

tal·i·pes
t. adductus
t. arcuatus
t. calcaneocavus
t. calcaneovalgocavus
t. calcaneovalgus
t. calcaneovarus
t. calcaneus
t. cavovalgus
t. cavus
t. equinovalgus
t. equinovarus
t. equinus
t. planovalgus
t. plantaris
t. planus
spasmodic t. planus
t. spasmodicus
t. transversoplanus
t. valgus
t. varus

tal·i·pom·a·nus

ta·lo·cal·ca·ne·al

ta·lo·cal·ca·ne·an

ta·lo·cru·ral

ta·lo·fib·u·lar

ta·lo·na·vic·u·lar

ta·lo·scaph·oid

ta·lo·tib·i·al

ta·lus *pl.* ta·li
    congenital vertical t.

tamp

tam·pon·ade

tap

Ta·pa·nol

Ta·par

tape
    adhesive t.
    Dacron t.
    Mersilene t.

Ta·per·loc hip pros·the·sis

TAR
    total ankle replacement

TAR (thrombocytopenia–
    absent radius) syn·drome

TARA
    total articular replacement
      arthroplasty

tar·sal

tar·sal·gia

tar·sa·lia

tar·sa·lis

tar·sec·to·my

tar·sec·to·pia

tar·soc·la·sis

tar·so·meg·a·ly

tar·so·meta·tar·sal

tar·so·pha·lan·ge·al

tar·sop·to·sis

tar·so·tar·sal

tar·so·tib·i·al

tar·sus
    bony t.

Tay·bi
    Rubinstein-T. syndrome

Tay·lor
    Girdlestone-T. procedure
    Gordon-T. amputation
    Jebson-T. hand function
      test
    Knight-T. orthosis
    Russell-T. interlocking
      nail system
    Russell-T. nail
    T. orthosis

Ta·zi·cef

Ta·zi·dime

TBI
    total body involved

T&C
    type and crossmatch

TCCK un·con·strained de·
    vice

TCO
    total contact orthosis

TCP
    tricalcium phosphate

Teale
    T's amputation
    T's operation

tear
    Bankart t.
    bucket-handle t.
    full-thickness t.
    meniscus t.
    parrot-beak meniscus t.
    partial-thickness t.

tear *(continued)*
    rotator cuff t.

Techne·Coll

Techne·Scan MDP

Techne·Scan PYP

tech·ne·ti·um
    t. Tc 99m oxidronate
    t. Tc 99m pyrophosphate
    t. Tc 99m (pyro- and tri-
        meta-) phosphates
    t. Tc 99m sulfur colloid

tech·nique
    Brooks t.
    Cobb-Lippman t.
    double-cementing t.
    four-ray t.
    Gibson t.
    Gillies and Millard t.
    Harri-Luque t.
    interlocking t.
    Miyakawa t.
    no-touch t.
    Orr t.
    posterolateral Gibson t.
    Rippstein II t.
    Roosevelt t.
    sleeve t.
    Strayer t.
    trap-door t.
    Trueta t.
    Vulpius t.

Tee·van
    T's law

Tef·lon

tei·no·dyn·ia

telo·phrag·ma

tem·plate
    femoral condyle t.
    tibial track t.

Tem·pra
    t. tendinum

te·nal·gia

ten·di·nes

ten·di·ni·tis
    bicipital t.
    calcific t.
    hypertrophic infiltrative t.
    t. ossificans traumatica
    quadriceps t.
    stenosing t.

ten·di·no·plas·ty

ten·di·no·su·ture

ten·di·nous

ten·do *pl.* ten·di·nes
    t. Achillis
    t. calcaneus
    t. conjunctivus

ten·dol·y·sis

ten·do·mu·cin

ten·don
    Achilles t.
    anterior tibial t.
    biceps t.
    calcaneal t.
    common t.
    conjoined t.
    extensor t.
    extensor carpi ulnaris t.
    extensor hallucis longus t.
    extensor pollicis brevis t.
    extensor pollicis longus t.
    flexor t.
    flexor carpi radialis t.
    flexor digitorum
        profundus t.
    flexor digitorum superfici-
        alis t.
    Galeazzi t. transfer
    gastrocnemius t.
    gracilis t.
    hamstring t.
    t. of Hector
    heel t.
    membranaceous t.
    patellar t., anterior
    patellar t., inferior

ten·don *(continued)*
    pes t.
    porous Dacron t.
    posterior tibial t.
    posterior tibialis t.
    pulled t.
    rectus femoris t.
    riders' t.
    rotator cuff t's
    semitendinosus t.
    snapping t.
    subscapularis t.
    supraspinatus t.
    triceps t.

ten·do·ni·tis

ten·don pass·er

ten·do·plas·ty

ten·do·syno·vi·tis

ten·do·vag·i·nal

ten·do·vag·i·ni·tis

te·nec·to·my

teno·de·sis

ten·odyn·ia

Ten·ol

ten·ol·y·sis

teno·my·ec·to·my

teno·myo·plas·ty

teno·my·ot·o·my

teno·nec·to·my

teno·ni·tis

ten·on·os·to·sis

ten·on·ta·gra

ten·on·ti·tis
    t. prolifera calcarea

ten·on·to·dyn·ia

ten·on·tog·ra·phy

ten·on·to·lem·mi·tis

ten·on·tol·o·gy

ten·on·to·myo·plas·ty

ten·on·to·my·ot·o·my

ten·on·to·phy·ma

ten·on·to·plas·ty

ten·on·to·the·ci·tis

teno·peri·os·ti·tis

teno·phyte

teno·plas·tic

teno·plas·ty

ten·or·rha·phy

teno·si·tis

ten·os·to·sis

teno·sus·pen·sion

teno·su·ture

teno·sy·ni·tis

teno·syn·o·vec·to·my

teno·syn·o·vi·tis
    t. acuta purulenta
    adhesive t.
    t. crepitans
    gonococcic t.
    gonorrheal t.
    granulomatous t.
    t. granulosa
    t. hypertrophica
    ossifying t.
    t. serosa chronica
    t. stenosans
    stenosing t.
    tuberculous t.
    villonodular t.
    villous t.

ten·ot·o·my

teno·vag·i·ni·tis

TENS
    transcutaneous electrical
      nerve stimulation

ten·sile load

ten·sion·ing
  graft t.

ten·sor
  t. fasciae latae

te·res
  t. major
  t. minor

Ter·ra·my·cin

Tesch·ler-Ni·co·la
  Killian and T.-N. syn-
    drome

test
  Adams forward bend t.
  Addis t.
  Allen's t.
  anterior apprehension t.
  antihuman globulin t.
  anvil t.
  Apley's t.
  Bekhterev's t.
  bench t.
  British t.
  Burns t.
  Callaway's t.
  Chiene t.
  Chilles squeeze t.
  clunk t.
  contralateral straight leg
    raising t.
  coordination extremity t.
  Crawford-Adams
    dexterity t.
  dexterity t.
  direct antihuman
    globulin t.
  direct Coombs' t.
  drop arm t.
  Dugas' t.
  Ely's t.
  external rotation recurva-
    tum t.
  Faber t.
  fadire t.
  femoral nerve stretch t.

test (continued)
  femoral nerve traction t.
  figure of 4 t.
  finger to toe t.
  flexion rotation drawer t.
  Fournier t.
  fulcrum t.
  Gaenslen's t
  glucose tolerance t.
  great toe extension t.
  grimace t.
  grind t.
  Hamilton's t.
  hemodynamic t.
  Hoover t.
  Hughston t.
  Hughston jerk t.
  indirect antihuman globu-
    lin t.
  indirect Coombs' t.
  Jacob shift t.
  Jansen's t.
  Jebsen-Taylor hand func-
    tion t.
  knee instability t.
  Kocher clamp t.
  Lachman t.
  latex agglutination t.
  MacIntosh t.
  Milgram t.
  Mills' t.
  Minnesota Rate of Manip-
    ulation T.
  Morton's t.
  nerve conduction t.
  noninvasive t.
  Noyes t.
  O'Connor finger
    dexterity t.
  Ober's t.
  patellar retraction t.
  Patrick's t.
  pelvic rock t.
  Phalen's t.
  pinprick t.
  pivot shift t.
  posterior drawer t.
  quadriceps t.

test *(continued)*
    quadriceps active t.
    RAAGG (rheumatoid ar-
        thritis agglutinin) t.
    reflex t.
    Romberg t.
    sagittal stress t.
    Schober t.
    Sharp-Purser t.
    Silfverskiöld t.
    Simmons t.
    Slocum's t.
    SLR (straight leg
        raising) t.
    Speed's t.
    sponge t.
    Spurling t.
    station t.
    straight leg raising t.
        (SLRT)
    Tensilon t.
    Thompson's t.
    thumb-nail t.
    tourniquet t.
    Trendelenburg's t.
    VonFrey hair t.
    Watson t.
    Wilson t.
    Yergason t.

test·er
    laxity t.
    Stryker/OSI laxity t.

test·ing
    cold t.
    physical t.
    pressure t.
    proprioceptive t.
    sensory t.

tet·ra·cy·cline

Tet·ra·cyn

tet·ra·ple·gia

tet·ra·ple·gic

Teu·fel
    T. orthosis

tex·tus *pl.* tex·tus
    t. connectivus collagenosus
    t. connectivus elasticus
    t. connectivus fibrosus
        compactus
    t. connectivus fibrosus la-
        mellaris
    t. muscularis
    t. muscularis nonstriatus
    t. muscularis striatus
    t. muscularis striatus car-
        diacus

TFL
    tensor fascia lata

T-frac·ture

TH
    thoracic

Th
    thigh
    thigh amputation

th
    thoracic

THA
    total hip arthroplasty

THARIES re·sur·fac·ing ar·
    thro·plas·ty

the·ca *pl.* the·cae
    t. medullare spinalis
    t. vertebralis

the·ci·tis

the·co·steg·no·sis

Thee·lin

the·nad

the·nal

the·nar

the·o·ry
    sliding filament t.

ther·a·pist
    physical t.
    registered occupational t.

ther·a·py
    occupational t.
    physical t.
    thrombolytic t.
    trigger-point t.

ther·mo·plas·tic

thi·a·zide

Thiele
    T. syndrome

Thie·mann
    T's disease
    T's syndrome

Thiersch
    Ollier-T. skin graft

thigh
    cricket t.

Tho·mas
    Mayo-T. collar
    T. collar
    T. heel
    T. procedure
    T. sign
    T. splint
    T., Thompson, and Straub
        procedure

Thomp·son
    Ferguson-T. osteotomy
    Royle-T. thumb adduction
    Thomas, T., and Straub
        procedure
    T. arthroplasty
    T. femoral head prosthesis
    T. hip prosthesis
    T. retractor
    T. telescoping V osteotomy
    T. test
    T., Parkridge, and Rich-
        ards total ankle replace-
        ment
    Whitman-T. procedure

Thom·son
    Rothmund-T. syndrome

tho·rac·ic

tho·rac·i·co·hu·mer·al

tho·raci·spi·nal

tho·ra·co·acro·mi·al

tho·ra·co·cyl·lo·sis

tho·ra·co·cyr·to·sis

tho·ra·co·dor·sal

tho·ra·co·lum·bar

tho·rax *pl.* tho·ra·ces
    barrel-shaped t.
    pyriform t.

Thorn·ton
    T. nail

THR
    total hip replacement

throm·bo·phle·bi·tis
    septic t.
    spinal t.

throm·bo·sis
    deep vein t.
    deep venous t. (DVT)
    venous t.

Throm·bo·stat

throm·bus *pl.* throm·bi

Throop
    Couch, DeRosa, and T.
        procedure

thryp·sis

thumb
    bifid t.
    bowler's t.
    gamekeeper's t.
    t. interphalangeal exten-
        sion assist
    t. ring
    spring swivel t.
    tennis t.
    trigger t.

thy·rox·in

TI
   tibia, complete (congenital
      absence of limb)

ti
   tibia, incomplete (congeni-
      tal absence of limb)

ti·a·pro·fen·ic acid

tib·ia
   t. antecurvata et valga
   saber t.
   saber-scabbard t.
   saber-shaped t.
   t. valga
   t. vara

tib·i·ad

tib·i·al

tib·i·a·le
   t. externum
   t. posticum

tib·i·al·gia

tib·i·a·lis
   t. anterior
   t. anticus
   t. posticus

tib·io·cal·ca·ne·an

tib·io·fem·or·al

tib·io·fib·u·lar

tib·io·na·vic·u·lar

tib·io·per·o·ne·al

tib·io·scaph·oid

tib·io·tar·sal

Ti·car

ti·car·cil·lin
   t. and clavulanate

Ti·choff
   T.-Linberg operation

Tiet·ze
   T's disease

Tiet·ze *(continued)*
   T's syndrome

Ti·khor
   T.-Linberg operation

Til·laux
   T.-Kleiger fracture

Till·man
   T. resurfacing procedure

time
   activated partial thrombo-
      plastin t.
   conduction t.
   double support t.
   partial thromboplastin t.
   prothrombin t.

Ti·men·tin

Tin·el
   T. sign

tip
   odontoid t.
   t. of sacral bone

tip plas·ty

Ti·rend

tir·ing

TIRR or·tho·sis

tis·sue
   bony t.
   cancellous t.
   compact t.
   connective t.
   cortical t.
   elastic t.
   fibrous t.
   myeloid t.
   osseous t.
   osteogenic t.
   osteoid t.
   skeletal t.

ti·ta·ni·um
   t. 6-4
   t. nitride

ti·ta·ni·um *(continued)*
    nitrided t. 6-4

TJ
    tendon jerk
    triceps jerk

TJR
    total joint replacement

TKA
    total knee arthroplasty

TKR
    total knee replacement

TLSO
    thoracolumbosacral or-
        thosis

TMJ
    temporomandibular joint

TNM stag·ing

TO
    thoracic orthosis

to·bra·my·cin

toe
    Biomet Total T.
    claw t.
    t. filler
    great t.
    hammer t.
    little t.
    mallet t.
    marathoner's t.
    pigeon t.
    tennis t.

toe-off

tog·gle

To·hen
    T. procedure

tol·met·in

to·mo·gram

to·mo·graph

to·mog·ra·phy
    computed t.
    computerized axial t.
    hypocycloidal t.
    single photon emission
        computed t. (SPECT)
    trispiral t.

to·mo·my·elog·ra·phy

tone
    muscle t.

tongs
    Crutchfield's t.
    Gardner-Wells t.
    skeletal t.
    Vinke t.

to·nus

Tooth
    Charcot-Marie-T. disease
    Marie-Charcot-T. disease

tooth *pl.* teeth
    t. of axis
    t. of epistropheus

to·pha·ceous

to·phus *pl.* to·phi

To·ron·to or·tho·sis

torque
    valgus t.

torr

tor·sion
    axial t.
    external tibial t.
    internal t.
    internal femoral t.
    lateral t.

tor·sion·al

tor·ti·col·lar

tor·ti·col·lis
    acute t.
    congenital t.
    dermatogenic t.

tor·ti·col·lis *(continued)*
    fixed t.
    intermittent t.
    mental t.
    myogenic t.
    paralytic t.
    rheumatoid t.
    spasmodic t.
    spastic t.
    spurious t.
    symptomatic t.

To·ta·cil·lin

To·tal Con·dy·lar semi·con·strained de·vice

tough·ness

tour·ni·quet
    pneumatic t.

Townes
    T. syndrome

Town·ley
    T. femur caliper
    T. tibial plateau plate
    T. unconstrained device

T-plas·ty

TPL-6 to·tal hip re·place·ment

TPR an·kle pros·the·sis

T-28 (Trapezoidal 28) pros·the·sis

tra·bec·u·la *pl.* tra·bec·u·lae
    trabeculae of bone

trac·er
    radioactive t.

tra·che·lo·cyl·lo·sis

tra·che·lo·cyr·to·sis

tra·che·lo·dyn·ia

tra·che·lo·ky·pho·sis

track·ing
    lateral t.

tract
    long t. of spinal cord
    Maissiat's t.
    pyramidal t. of spinal cord
    spinal t. of trigeminal
      nerve

trac·tion
    90-90 t.
    axial t.
    balanced t.
    Bryant's t.
    Buck's t.
    Buck's extension t.
    cervical t.
    Cotrel t.
    Crutchfield's skeletal t.
    Dunlop t.
    elastic t.
    elastic finger t.
    floating t.
    halo t.
    halo-femoral t.
    halo-pelvic t.
    Hare t.
    K-wire skeletal t.
    lumbar t.
    Lyman-Smith t.
    Neufeld roller t.
    overhead t.
    pelvic t.
    plaster t.
    Quigley t.
    Russell t.
    sidearm skin t.
    skeletal t.
    skin t.
    suspended t.
    tibial pin t.
    transverse t.
    vertebral t.
    weight t.
    well-leg t.
    windlass t.

trac·tus *pl.* trac·tus
    t. iliotibialis
    t. iliotibialis [Maissiati]

trag·o·po·dia

train·ing
    gait t.

trans·cap·i·tate

trans·con·dy·loid

trans·cor·ti·cal

tran·sect

trans·fer
    Baker tendon t.
    Bunnell tendon t.
    Chandler tendon t.
    double toe t.
    dynamic tendon t.
    Eggers tendon t.
    Galeazzi tendon t.
    iliopsoas t.
    Kelikian tendon t.
    medial tibial tubercle t.
    muscle t.
    Mustard iliopsoas t.
    second toe microvascular t.
    Sharrard iliopsoas t.
    static hand tendon t.
    static tendon t.
    Sutherland tendon t.
    Tachdjian tendon t.
    tendon t.
    toe phalanx t.

trans·glen·oid

trans·ham·ate

trans·is·chi·al
    cervicothoracic t.

trans·la·tion
    anteroposterior t.
    mediolateral t.

trans·lu·cent

trans·meta·tar·sal

trans·pe·dic·u·lar

trans·plant
    bone marrow t.
    Hauser t.

trans·plan·tar

trans·plan·ta·tion
    tendon t.

trans·ra·di·al

trans·sa·cral

trans·scaph·oid

trans·sy·no·vi·al

Trans·tib·i·al drill guide sys·tem

trans·tri·que·tral

trans·ver·sec·to·my

trans·ver·so·cos·tal

trans·ver·sot·o·my

tra·pe·zi·ec·to·my

tra·pe·zio·cap·i·tate

tra·pe·zio·meta·car·pal

tra·pe·zio·scaph·oid

tra·pe·zio·trap·e·zoid

tra·pe·zi·um

tra·pe·zi·us

Tra·pe·zoi·dal 28 (T-28) pros·the·sis

trap·ping
    Conrad-Bugg t.

trau·ma *pl.* trau·mas, trau·ma·ta

Traut·man Lock·tite hook

tray
    tibial t.

treat·ment
  hydrotherapy t.
  infrared t.
  Kittel's t.
  Klapp's creeping t.
  Lerich's t.
  Orr t.
  Paul's t.
  salicyl t.
  Trueta t.

trem·or

Tre·nau·nay
  Klippel-T.-Weber syn-
    drome

Tren·dar

Tren·del·en·burg
  T. sign
  T's symptom
  T's test

Tren·ta·ni
  Paltrinieri-T. resurfacing
    procedure
  Sharrard-T. resurfacing
    procedure

tre·phine

trep·pe

Tre·vor
  T's disease

tri·ad
  t. of skeletal muscle

tri·an·gle
  Alsberg's t.
  clavipectoral t.
  Codman's t.
  t. of elbow
  Kager's t.
  Kanavel's t.
  t's of neck
  popliteal t. of femur
  sacral t.
  von Weber's t.
  Ward's t.

Tri-Ax·i·al el·bow pros·the·
  sis

Tri·az·ole

tri·bol·o·gy

tri·cal·ci·um phos·phate

tri·ceps
  t. surae

tri·chlo·ro·ace·tic acid

trich·ter·brust

tri·cip·i·tal

tri·cor·ti·cate

tri·eth·yl·amine
  t. salicylate

tri·gas·tric

tri·go·num *pl.* tri·go·na
  t. clavipectorale
  t. deltoideopectorale
  t. omoclaviculare

Trik·acide

Tril·lat
  Elmslie-T. method
  Elmslie-T. procedure
  T. procedure

Tri·lock fem·or·al com·po·
  nent

tri·meth·o·prim
  sulfamethoxazole and t.

Trin·kle
  T. brace

tri·pha·lan·ge·al

tri·pha·lan·gia

tri·pha·lan·gism

Trip·ier
  T's amputation

tri·que·tral

tri·que·trous

tri·que·trum

Tri·sul·fam

Triz·ma buf·fer

tro·car
    blunt t.

tro·chan·ter
    greater t.
    lesser t.
    t. major
    t. minor
    rudimentary t.
    small t.
    t. tertius

tro·chan·ter·i·an

tro·chan·ter·ic

tro·chan·ter·itis

tro·chan·ter·plas·ty

tro·chan·tin

tro·chan·tin·i·an

troch·i·ter

troch·i·te·ri·an

troch·lea
    t. fibularis calcanei
    t. humeri
    t. of humerus
    muscular t.
    t. muscularis
    peroneal t. of calcaneus
    t. peronealis calcanei
    t. phalangis digitorum
        manus
    t. phalangis digitorum
        pedis
    t. tali
    t. of talus

tro·choi·des

tro·pism
    facet t.

tro·po·col·la·gen

Tru-Cut nee·dle

Tru·e·ta
    T. method
    T. technique
    T. treatment

Trum·ble
    T. arthrodesis

Trüm·mer·feld
    T. line

trun·cate

T&S
    type and screen

TSA
    total shoulder arthroplasty

TSC
    technetium sulfur colloid

TSH
    thyroid-stimulating hor-
        mone

Tsu·ge
    T. tendon repair

TTAP
    threaded titanium acetab-
        ular prosthesis

T-28 to·tal hip re·place·ment

tube
    Dacron t.
    exchange t.

tu·ber pl. tu·bers, tu·be·ra
    t. calcanei
    iliopubic t.
    t. ischiadicum
    t. ischiale
    t. radii
    t. of radius
    sciatic t.

tu·ber·cle
    adductor t.
    adductor t. of femur
    t. of anterior scalene mus-
        cle
    anterior tibial t.

tu·ber·cle *(continued)*
    t. of atlas, anterior
    t. of atlas, posterior
    brachial t. of humerus
    calcaneal t.
    carotid t.
    cervical t's
    t. of cervical vertebrae, anterior
    t. of cervical vertebrae, posterior
    Chaput t.
    Chassaignac's t.
    conoid t.
    deltoid t.
    dorsal t. of radius
    t. of fibula, posterior
    Gerdy's t.
    greater t. of calcaneus
    t. of greater multangular bone
    t. of humerus
    t. of humerus, anterior, of Meckel
    t. of humerus, anterior, of Weber
    t. of humerus, external
    t. of humerus, greater
    t. of humerus, internal
    t. of humerus, lesser
    t. of humerus, posterior
    iliac t.
    iliopectineal t.
    iliopubic t.
    inferior t. of Humphrey
    infraglenoid t.
    intercondylar t.
    intercondylar t., lateral
    intercondylar t., medial
    lesser t. of calcaneus
    Lisfranc's t.
    Lister's t.
    mamillary t.
    muscular t. of atlas
    t. of navicular bone
    nuchal t.
    obturator t., anterior
    obturator t., posterior

tu·ber·cle *(continued)*
    plantar t.
    t. of posterior process of talus, lateral
    t. of posterior process of talus, medial
    pubic t. of pubic bone
    t. of rib
    scalene t.
    t. of scaphoid bone
    t. of sixth cervical vertebra, anterior
    t. of sixth cervical vertebra, carotid
    t. of sixth cervical vertebra, posterior
    superior t. of Henle
    superior t. of Humphrey
    supraglenoid t.
    t. of tibia
    tibial t.
    t. of Tillaux-Chaput
    transverse t. of fourth tarsal bone
    t. of trapezium
    trochanteric t.
    t. of ulna
    t's of vertebra

tu·ber·cu·lo·sis
    t. of bones and joints
    skeletal t.
    spinal t.
    t. of spine

tu·ber·cu·lum *pl.* tu·ber·cu·la
    t. adductorium femoris
    t. anterius atlantis
    t. anterius vertebrae cervicalis sextae
    t. anterius vertebrarum cervicalium
    t. arthriticum
    t. calcanei
    t. caroticum vertebrae cervicalis sextae
    t. conoideum
    t. costae

tu·ber·cu·lum *(continued)*
  t. dolorosum
  t. iliacum
  t. infraglenoidale
  t. intercondylare laterale
  t. intercondylare mediale
  t. intercondyloideum
  t. intercondyloideum laterale
  t. intercondyloideum mediale
  t. laterale processus posterioris tali
  t. majus humeri
  t. mediale processus posterioris tali
  t. minus humeri
  t. musculi scaleni anterioris
  t. obturatorium anterius
  t. obturatorium posterius
  t. ossis multanguli majoris
  t. ossis navicularis
  t. ossis scaphoidei
  t. ossis trapezii
  t. posterius atlantis
  t. posterius vertebrae cervicalis sextae
  t. posterius vertebrarum cervicalium
  t. pubicum ossis pubis
  t. scaleni [Lisfranci]
  t. supraglenoidale

tu·be·ros·i·tas *pl.* tu·be·ro·si·ta·tes
  t. coracoidea
  t. costae II
  t. costalis claviculae
  t. deltoidea humeri
  t. femoris externa
  t. femoris interna
  t. glutea femoris
  t. iliaca
  t. infraglenoidalis
  t. musculi serrati anterioris
  t. ossis cuboidei

tu·be·ros·i·tas *(continued)*
  t. ossis metatarsalis primi
  t. ossis metatarsalis quinti
  t. ossis navicularis
  t. patellaris
  t. phalangis distalis manus
  t. phalangis distalis pedis
  t. radii
  t. sacralis
  t. supraglenoidalis scapulae
  t. tibiae
  t. tibiae externa
  t. tibiae interna
  t. ulnae
  t. unguicularis manus
  t. unguicularis pedis

tu·be·ros·i·ty
  adductor t.
  t. for anterior serratus muscle
  biceps t.
  bicipital t.
  t. of calcaneus
  t. of clavicle
  coracoid t.
  costal t. of clavicle
  t. of cuboid bone
  deltoid t. of humerus
  distal t. of fingers
  distal t. of toes
  t. of femur, external
  t. of femur, internal
  t. of femur, lateral
  t. of femur, medial
  t. of fifth metatarsal
  t. of first carpal bone
  t. of first metatarsal
  t. of fourth tarsal bone
  gluteal t. of femur
  greater t. of humerus
  t. of greater multangular bone
  t's of humerus
  iliac t.
  infraglenoid t.

tu·be·ros·i·ty *(continued)*
    ischial t.
    t. of ischium
    lesser t. of humerus
    t. of navicular bone
    patellar t.
    t. of pubic bone
    radial t.
    t. of radius
    sacral t.
    t. of scaphoid bone
    scapular t. of Henle
    t. of second rib
    t. for serratus anterior
      muscle
    supraglenoid t.
    t. of tibia
    t. of tibia, external
    t. of tibia, internal
    t. of trapezium
    t. of ulna
    unguicular t.

tub·ing
    medullary vent t.

tu·bule
    T t's
    transverse t.

tuft
    synovial t's

tu·me·fac·tion

tu·mor
    bone t.
    bone cell t.
    brown t.
    cartilage t.
    Codman's t.
    desmoid t.
    Ewing's t.
    giant cell t.
    glomus t.
    Hodgkin t.
    intramedullary t.
    march t.
    osseous t.
    primary t. of bone

tu·mor *(continued)*
    round cell t.
    Schwann t.
    Steiner's t's
    white t.

tun·nel
    carpal t.
    cubital t.
    femoral t.
    flexor t.
    tarsal t.
    tibial t.

Tup·per
    T. arthroplasty

Tur·co
    T. procedure

tur·gid

Tur·ner
    Aufranc-T. total hip re-
      placement
    Parsonage-T. syndrome
    T's syndrome

turn·over
    bone t.

Tu·ryn
    T. sign

T1-weight·ed image

T2-weight·ed image

twist·er
    wire t.

twitch
    fast t.
    slow t.

TWZ
    triangular working zone

TX
    traction
    transplant

TXN
    traction

Ty·cron su·ture

Ty·le·nol

ty·lo·ma

type

    Dejerine-Landouzy t.
    Duchenne's t.
    Duchenne-Landouzy t.
    Erb-Zimmerlin t.

type *(continued)*

    Landouzy's t.
    Landouzy-Dejerine t.
    Leyden-Möbius t.
    Simmerlin t.
    storiform-pleomorphic t.
    Zimmerlin's t.

typ·ing

    bone t.

U
    ulna, complete (congenital
        absence of limb)

u
    ulna, incomplete (congeni-
        tal absence of limb)

UA
    urinalysis

uar·thri·tis

UC-BL (University of
    California Biomechanics
    Laboratory) in·sert

UCB or·tho·sis

UCI un·con·strained de·vice

UHMWPE
    ultrahigh molecular
        weight polyethylene

ul·cer
    amputating u.
    decubitus u.
    gouty u.

Ull·mann
    U's line

ul·na pl. ul·nae

ul·nad

ul·nar

ul·na·re

ul·na·ris

ul·nen

ul·no·car·pal

ul·no·ra·di·al

ul·ti·mi·ster·nal

ul·ti·mum mo·ri·ens

Ul·tra·cef

Ul·tra·coat

un·car·thro·sis

un·ci·for·me

un·ci·nal

un·ci·nate

un·ci·na·tum

un·co·ver·te·bral

un·cus
    u. corporis
    u. of hamate bone

un·der·toe

un·guis pl. un·gues
    u. incarnatus

uni·ar·tic·u·lar

uni·ceps

uni·com·part·men·tal

Uni·flex nail

Uni·gen

uni·lat·er·al

un·ion
    delayed u.
    faulty u.
    secondary u.
    vicious u.

uni·por·tal

unit
    basic multicellular u.
    cervicocranial u.
    functional spinal u.
    quick-change wrist u.
    rotator u.
    standard constant friction
        wrist u.
    torsion u.
    wrist u.

unit *(continued)*
　　wrist flexion u.

Uni·ver·sal rod

Uni·ver·si·ty of Cal·i·for·
　　nia, Ir·vine, to·tal an·kle
　　re·place·ment

up·bit·ing

up·right

up·take
　　osseous u.

Ura·cel

urar·thri·tis

urat·ic

uric acid

uri·case

uri·nal·y·sis

Uro·plus

U.S. re·trac·tor

va·gi·na *pl.* va·gi·nae
 v. communis musculorum
 flexorum
 v. femoris
 vaginae fibrosae digitorum
 manus
 vaginae fibrosae digitorum
 pedis
 v. fibrosa tendinis
 vaginae mucosae
 v. mucosa tendinis
 v. musculorum fibularium
 communis
 v. musculorum peroneo-
 rum communis
 vaginae synoviales
 v. synovialis communis
 musculorum flexorum
 vaginae synoviales digitorum manus
 vaginae synoviales digitorum pedis
 v. synovialis intertubercu-
 laris
 v. synovialis musculorum
 fibularium communis
 v. synovialis musculi obliqui superioris
 v. synovialis musculorum
 peroneorum communis
 v. synovialis tendinis
 vaginae synoviales ten-
 dinum digitorum manus
 vaginae synoviales ten-
 dinum digitorum pedis
 v. synovialis tendinis musculi flexoris carpi radialis
 v. synovialis tendinis musculi flexoris hallucis
 longi
 v. synovialis tendinis musculi tibialis posterioris
 v. tendinis

va·gi·na *(continued)*
 vaginae tendinum digito-
 rum manus
 vaginae tendinum digito-
 rum pedis
 v. tendinum musculorum
 abductoris longi et extensoris brevis pollicis
 v. tendinum musculorum
 extensorum carpi radi-
 alium
 v. tendinis musculi extensoris carpi ulnaris
 v. tendinum musculorum
 extensoris digitorum
 communis et extensoris
 v. tendinum musculorum
 extensoris digitorum et
 extensoris indicis
 v. tendinis musculi extensoris digiti minimi
 vaginae tendinum musculi
 extensoris digitorum
 pedis longi
 v. tendinis musculi extensoris hallucis longi
 v. tendinis musculi extensoris pollicis longi
 v. tendinis musculi fibularis longi plantaris
 v. tendinis musculi flexoris
 carpi radialis
 vaginae tendinum musculi
 flexoris digitorum pedis
 longi
 v. tendinis musculi flexoris
 hallucis longi
 v. tendinis musculi flexoris
 pollicis longi
 v. tendinis musculi obliqui
 superioris
 v. tendinis musculi pero-
 nei longi plantaris

va·gi·na *(continued)*
 v. tendinis musculi tibialis
  anterioris
 v. tendinis musculi tibialis
  posterioris

Vai·nio
 V. arthroplasty

Val·a·dol

Val·er·gen-10

Val·er·gen-20

val·gus
 forefoot v.

Valls
 V. hip prosthesis

Val·or·in

Val·par com·po·nent work
 sam·ple se·ries

Val·sal·va
 V's maneuver

van Bu·chem
 van B's syndrome

Van·cer·il

van Ness
 Broggreve-van N. rotation
  osteotomy
 van N. rotation

Van·zet·ti
 V. sign

Vari·kopf
 V. total hip replacement

var·us
 forefoot v.

vas·cu·lar

vaso·con·stric·tion

vaso·di·la·tion

vaso·spas·tic

vas·tus
 v. lateralis
 v. medialis

VATER
 vertebral defects, anal
  atresia, tracheoesopha-
  geal fistula with esopha-
  geal atresia, and radial
  and renal anomalies

VATER as·so·ci·a·tion

VDDR
 vitamin D–dependent
  rickets

VDRR
 vitamin D–resistant rickets

vec·tor

vein
 axillary v.
 basilic v.
 brachial v's
 cephalic v.
 femoral v.
 jugular v.
 median basilic v.
 median cephalic v.
 popliteal v.
 posterior tibial v.
 radial v's
 saphenous v.
 segmental v.
 subclavian v.

Vel·cro splint

Ve·le·a·nu
 V., Rosianu, and Ionescu
  procedure

ve·loc·i·ty
 average v.
 average angular v.
 foot v.
 walking v.

Vel·o·sef

Vel·peau
 V's deformity
 V. dressing

ve·no·gram

ve·nog·ra·phy
    intraosseous v.

ven·ter *pl.* ven·tres
    v. ilii
    v. scapulae

ven·tral

ven·ule

Ver·dan
    V. grafts and flaps
    V. pollicization
    V. tendon repair

Ver·neuil
    V's disease

ver·ru·ca *pl.* ver·ru·cae

Verse
    V's disease

ver·te·bra *pl.* ver·te·brae
    abdominal vertebrae
    balanced v.
    basilar v.
    butterfly v.
    caudal vertebrae
    caudate vertebrae
    cervical vertebrae
    vertebrae cervicales
    cleft v.
    vertebrae coccygeae
    coccygeal vertebrae
    codfish v.
    vertebrae colli
    v. dentata
    dorsal vertebrae
    false vertebrae
    H v.
    ivory v.
    vertebrae lumbales
    lumbar vertebrae
    v. magnum
    movable v.
    odontoid v.
    olisthetic v.
    picture frame v.
    v. plana

ver·te·bra *(continued)*
    v. prominens
    prominent v.
    sacral vertebrae
    vertebrae sacrales
    sternal v.
    supernumerary vertebrae
    terminal v., great
    vertebrae thoracales
    thoracic vertebrae
    vertebrae thoracicae
    transitional v.
    true vertebrae

ver·te·bral

ver·te·brar·i·um

ver·te·brec·to·my

ver·te·bro·chon·dral

ver·te·bro·cos·tal

ver·te·bro·fem·or·al

ver·te·bro·gen·ic

ver·te·bro·il·i·ac

ver·te·bro·sa·cral

ver·te·bro·ster·nal

ver·ti·cal

ve·sa·li·a·num

Ve·sa·li·us
    ligament of V.

ves·i·cle
    matrix v's

ves·sel
    blood v.
    subsynovial retinacular v's

vest
    halo v.

ves·tig·i·al

Ve·ze·ri·dis
    Karkousis and V. proce-
      dure

VI
valgus index

vi·a·ble

Vi·bra·my·cin

Vi·bra-Tabs

Vi·cryl su·ture

Vi·dal
V.-Ardrey fixation device

view
Alexander's v.
apical v.
apical lordotic v.
apical oblique v.
axial v.
axillary v.
ball-catcher's v.
Breuerton v.
Carter-Rowe v.
clenched fist v.
coned-down v.
Ferguson v.
flexion weight-bearing v.
frog-leg lateral v.
Grashey v.
Hobb v.
Hugston v.
lateral v.
Merchant v.
mortise v.
Neer lateral v.
Neer transscapular v.
neutral-flexion-
extension v.
Norgaard v.
open-mouth v.
plantar axial v. of foot
push-pull ankle stress v.
radial head-capitellar v.
sagittal extension v.
sagittal flexion v.
scapular Y v.
serendipity v.
Stagnara v.
sunset v.
tangential v.

view *(continued)*
true lateral v.
tunnel v.
von Rosen v.

vig·o·rim·e·ter
Martin v.

vil·lo·nod·u·lar

vil·lus *pl.* vil·li
synovial villi
villi synoviales

vil·lus·ec·to·my

vi·men·tin

vin·cu·lum *pl.* vin·cu·la
v. breve
v. longum
vincula tendinum digito-
rum manus
vincula tendinum digito-
rum pedis
vincula of tendons of fingers
vincula of tendons of toes

Vinke
V. tongs

vis·cero·skel·e·tal

vis·co·elas·tic·i·ty

VISI
volar flexed intercalated
segment instability

Vi·tal
Hoffman-V. fixation device

Vi·tal·li·um

vi·ta·min
v. D

Vlad·i·mir·off
V. operation
V.-Mikulicz amputation

VMO
vastus medialis obliquus

vo·la *pl.* vo·lae
    v. manus
    v. pedis

vo·lar

vo·lar·dor·sal

vo·la·ris

Volk·mann
    V's canals
    V's contracture
    V's deformity
    V's disease
    V. fracture
    V's ischemia
    V. rake retractor
    V's subluxation
    V's syndrome

Vol·kov
    V.-Oganesyan fixation device

vol·ume
    blood v.
    cell v.
    mean corpuscular v.

Volz
    V. arthroplasty
    V. prosthesis

von Bahr
    von B. screw

VonFrey
    VonF. hair test

von Gies
    von G. joint

von Rosen
    von R. splint
    von R. view

von We·ber
    von W's triangle

Voor·hoeve
    V's disease

Vro·lik
    V's disease

VSP
    spinal fusion implant

Vul·pi·us
    V. procedure
    V. technique
    V.-Compere procedure

V-Y plas·ty

V-Y quad·ri·ceps·plas·ty

Waal·er
  Rose-W. test

Waar·den·burg
  W's syndrome

Wac·ken·heim
  W's basilar line
  W's line

Wads·worth
  W. elbow prosthesis

Wag·ner
  W. arthroplasty
  W. fixation device
  W. incision
  W's line
  W. procedure
  W. prosthesis
  W. resurfacing hip arthro-
    plasty
  W. resurfacing procedure
  W. tendon advancement

Wag·staffe
  W's fracture

Wal·den·ström
  W's disease

walk

Walk·er
  Pritchard-W. elbow pros-
    thesis

walk·er
  Cam w.

walk·ing
  heel w.
  toe w.

Wall·dius
  W. fully constrained de-
    vice

Wal·ther
  W's oblique ligament

Wan·gen·steen
  W. needle holder

Ward
  W's triangle

War·ner
  W. and Farber procedure

wart
  plantar w.

War·ten·berg
  W's disease
  W. sign

wash·er
  C-w.
  narrow w.
  soft-tissue w.
  spiked w.
  suture w.
  wide w.

Was·ser·stein
  W. fixation device

Wat·son
  W. test
  W.-Jones arthrodesis
  W.-Jones procedure

Waugh
  W. unconstrained device

WBAT
  weight bearing as toler-
    ated

WBC
  white blood cell

wbc
  white blood cell

WD
  wrist disarticulation

Weav·er
  W. syndrome
  W. and Dunn procedure

Webb
    Gristina and W. prosthesis
    W. bolt

Web·er
    anterior tubercle of hu-
        merus of W.
    common ligament of knee
        (of W.)
    Klippel-Trenaunay-W.
        syndrome
    W. fracture
    W's zone

Web·ril

web space plas·ty

wedge
    w. in cast
    closing w.
    medial heel w.
    tibial w.

wedg·ing
    w. of vertebra

Weg·ner
    W's disease
    W. line

Weh·gen

Wei·gert
    W's iron hematoxylin solu-
        tion

weight
    modular w's

weight-bear·ing
    protected w.-b.

Weill
    Leri-W. dyschondrosteosis
    W.-Marchesani syndrome

Wein·stein
    Simms-W. monofilament

Weiss
    Chvostek-W. sign
    W. sign
    W. spring

Weiss·mann
    W's bundle
    W's fibers

Weit·brecht
    ligament of antibrachium
        (of W.)
    prismatic ligament of W.
    W's cartilage
    W's cord
    W's foramen
    W's ligament
    W's retinaculum

Weit·lan·er
    W. retractor

Wells
    Gardner-W. calipers
    Gardner-W. tongs
    Hay-W. syndrome

Wer·ner
    W's syndrome

WEST
    work evaluation systems
        technology

West
    W. and Soto-Hall proce-
        dure

whip·lash

whirl·pool

whisk·er·ing

White
    Gill, Manning, and W.
        lumbar spinal fusion
    W. arthrodesis
    W. procedure
    W. slide procedure

White·cloud
    W. and Larocca spinal fu-
        sion

White·side
    W. semiconstrained device

whit·low
  herpetic w.

Whit·man
  W. frame
  W. osteotomy
  W. plate
  W. procedure
  W. talectomy
  W.-Thompson procedure

WHO
  wrist-hand orthosis

whorl
  bone w.

Wi·berg
  W. patellar shape
  W. shelf procedure

Wick·strom
  W. arthrodesis

Wil·li
  Prader-W. syndrome

Wil·liams
  W. flexion exercise
  W. orthosis
  W. syndrome

Wil·lis
  Kickaldy and W. arthro-
    desis

Wills
  Brooker-W. nail

Wil·ming·ton
  W. brace
  W. jacket

Wilms
  aniridia–W. tumor associ-
    ation

Wil·son
  Amstutz and W. osteotomy
  Compare and W. fusion
  W. arthrodesis
  W's disease
  W. graft
  W. plate

Wil·son *(continued)*
  W. procedure
  W. test
  W.-Burstein total hip re-
    placement
  W. and Jacobs procedure
  W. and McKeever proce-
    dure

Win·ber·ger
  W. line

win·dow
  cortical subcrestal w.

wing
  w. of ilium
  lateral w. of sacrum

Wing·field
  W. frame

Win·o·grad
  W. procedure

Win·quist
  W. classification (for com-
    minution of femoral frac-
    ture)
  W.-Hansen classification
    (for comminution of fem-
    oral fractures)

Wins·low
  W's ligament

wire
  Bunnell pull out w.
  guide w.
  K-w.
  Kirschner w.
  spinous process w.
  threaded w.

wire twist·er
  Shifrin w.t.

wir·ing
  cerclage w.
  interspinous w.
  sublaminar w.

Wis·sin·ger
  W. rod

Wolf
    W. procedure

Wolfe
    Krause-W. skin graft
    W. skin graft
    W.-graft flap

Wolff
    W's law

Wood·ruff
    W. screw

Wood·son
    W. dissector
    W. elevator

Wood·ward
    W. procedure

work
    w. conditioning
    w. hardening

work eval·u·a·tion sys·tem
    tech·nol·o·gy

wrench
    cannulated w.
    flat w.
    Harrington w.
    hex w.

Wright
    W. unconstrained device

Wris·berg
    Henry and W. ligament
    W's ligament

wrist
    Arizona w.
    SLAC (scapholunate ad-
        vanced collapse) w.
    tennis w.

wrist unit
    quick-change w.u.
    standard constant friction
        w.u.

wry·neck

Wy·cil·lin

xan·tho·ma
  malignant fibrous x.

xeno·graft
  bovine x.

xiphi·ster·nal

xiphi·ster·num

xipho·cos·tal

xiph·odyn·ia

xiph·oid

xiph·oi·di·tis

XS
  xiphisternum

xy·phoid

Y car·ti·lage

Yer·ga·son
Y. test

Y frac·ture

YIS un·con·strained de·vice

Y lig·a·ment

Y-line

Y-os·te·ot·o·my

Young
Y. procedure

Yuan
Y. I plate
Y. plate

Za·dik
　Z. procedure

Zan·tac

Zar·ins
　Z. and Rowe procedure

Zef·a·zone

Zeir
　Z. procedure

Zell·weg·er
　Z. syndrome

Zen·ker
　Z's degeneration
　Z's necrosis

Zen·o·tech

Zick·el
　Z. fracture
　Z. nail

Ziel·ke
　Z. instrumentation
　Z. sacral bar
　Z. spinal fusion implant

Zim·mer
　Z. compression hip screw
　Z. femoral condyle blade
　　plate
　Z. shoulder prosthesis
　Z. tibia bolt

Zim·mer·lin
　Z's type

Zin·a·cef

Z-leng·then·ing

ZMS in·tra·med·ul·lary fix·
　a·tion sys·tem

Zol·i·cef

zo·na *pl.* zo·nae
　z. orbicularis articulationis
　　coxae
　z. Weberi

zone
　Charnley z.
　cut-back z.
　DeLee z.
　Kambin's triangular work-
　　ing z.
　McNab's hidden z.
　orbicular z. of hip joint
　z. of transition
　triangular working z.
　Weber's z.

Z-plas·ty

Zuel·zer
　Z. hood

zy·ga·po·phys·e·al

zy·ga·poph·y·sis *pl.* zy·ga·
　poph·y·ses

zy·go·style